Yoga Therapy
Theory

Yoga Therapy Theory

MODERN METHODS BASED ON TRADITIONAL TEACHINGS OF HUMAN STRUCTURE AND FUNCTION

Kazuo Keishin Kimura

Translated by Madoka Onizuka Chase

Copyright © 2016 Japan Yoga Niketan.
All rights reserved.
This book is not intended as a substitute for the medical advice of physicians. The reader should consult a physician in matters relating to his/her health and particularly with respect to any symptoms that may require diagnosis or medical attention.
To inquire regarding reproduction of this book in part or in whole, please contact:
Japan Yoga Niketan
1-2-24 Sanbonmatsu
Yonago-shi, Tottori
Japan 683-0842
E-mail: yoganiketan@yoganiketan.jp
Tel: +81-859-22-3503 Fax: +81-859-22-1446

ISBN: 1536906263
ISBN 13: 9781536906264

Contents

Acknowledgments ix

Introduction xi
1) Yoga Today xi
2) Purpose of this Book. xiii
3) What Causes Illness? xiii
4) My First Encounters with Yoga Therapy. xiv
5) Theories of Human Structure and Function. xvi
6) Yoga Therapy and Ayurveda. xviii
7) The Japan Yoga Therapy Society (JYTS) xix

Part I   **Yoga Therapy Theory: Theories of Human
Structure and Function** 1

Chapter 1 What is Yoga Therapy?. 3
1) The Role of Yoga Therapists 3
2) The Difference Between Yoga Instructors
and Yoga Therapists 5
3) Ayurveda: India's Traditional Medicine. 7
4) Three Categories of Yoga Therapy Techniques 12

Chapter 2 Yoga's Theory of Human Structure and its
Application to Stress Management. 18
1) The Theory of Human Structure as Written in
the *Taittiriya Upanishad* (Pancha Kosha Theory). 19
2) The *Katha Upanishad* "Human Chariot Theory" 24
3) Human Functions as Explained in the
Pancha Kosha and Human Chariot Theories 29

	4)	Ayurveda's Human Structure and Function Theories as Seen in the *Charaka Samhita* 32
	5)	The Role of Physicians as Explained in the *Charaka Samhita* 41

Part II   **Yoga Therapy in Practice: Yoga Therapy Assessment (YTA)**. 47

Chapter 1   Yoga Therapy Principles for Assessment and Instruction. . . 49

      1)   The Six Stages in Yoga Therapy. 49

Chapter 2   Discerning the Unreal from the Real and Yoga Therapy Assessment (YTA). 58

      1)   Yoga Therapy Assessment (YTA) and Patanjali's *Yoga Sutras* 59

      2)   Yoga Therapy Assessment (YTA) and The *Bhagavad Gita* 66

      3)   Yoga Therapy Assessment (YTA) and Ayurvedic Assessment. 70

      4)   Yoga Therapy Assessment (YTA) and Counseling Skills 72

Part III   **The Koshas: Yoga Therapy Assessment (YTA) and Yoga Therapy Instruction (YTI)** 73

Chapter 1   Yoga Therapy Assessment (YTA) and Yoga Therapy Instruction (YTI) for the Annamaya Kosha 75

      1)   Yoga Therapy's Pathogenesis Theory and the Annamaya Kosha 75

      2)   Yoga Therapy Assessment (YTA) of the Annamaya Kosha 76

      3)   Ayurveda-Based Yoga Therapy Assessment. 78

      4)   Principles of Yoga Therapy Instruction (YTI) for the Annamaya Kosha 83

      5)   Prevention of Adverse Events in the Annamaya Kosha 117

      6)   Fictional Case Studies: Annamaya Kosha 119

Chapter 2 Yoga Therapy Assessment (YTA) and Yoga Therapy Instruction (YTI) for the Pranamaya Kosha 128

1) Yoga Therapy's Pathogenesis Theory and the Pranamaya Kosha 128

2) Yoga Therapy Assessment (YTA) of the Pranamaya Kosha 129

3) Principles of Yoga Therapy Instruction (YTI) for the Pranamaya Kosha 130

4) Prevention of Adverse Events in the Pranamaya Kosha 132

5) Physiological Changes and Pranayama 133

6) Fictional Case Studies: Pranamaya Kosha 140

Chapter 3 Yoga Therapy Assessment (YTA) and Yoga Therapy Instruction (YTI) for the Manomaya Kosha 148

1) Yoga Therapy's Pathogenesis Theory and the Manomaya Kosha 148

2) Yoga Therapy Assessment (YTA) and the Manomaya Kosha 149

3) Principles of Yoga Therapy Instruction (YTI) and the Manomaya Kosha 151

4) Prevention of Adverse Events in the Manomaya Kosha 157

5) How Changes in the Manomaya Kosha Can Manifest as Physiological Changes 158

6) Fictional Case Studies: Manomaya Kosha 160

Chapter 4 Yoga Therapy Assessment (YTA) and Yoga Therapy Instruction (YTI) For The Vijnanamaya Kosha: Addressing Functions of the Buddhi and Forgotten Memories 170

1) Yoga Therapy's Pathogenesis Theory and the Vijnanamaya Kosha. 170

2) Yoga Therapy Assessment (YTA) and the Vijnanamaya Kosha 171

3) Principles of Yoga Therapy Instruction (YTI) for the Vijnanamaya Kosha. 187

4) Purification of and Instruction for the Vijnanamaya Kosha. 189

5) Prevention of Adverse Events in the Vijnanamaya Kosha. 199

6) Fictional Case Studies: Vijnanamaya Kosha 200

Chapter 5 Yoga Therapy Assessment (YTA) and Yoga Therapy Instruction (YTI) for the Anandamaya Kosha: Addressing Forgotten Memories, the Ahamkara and Chitta 208

1) Yoga Therapy's Pathogenesis Theory and the Anandamaya Kosha. 208

2) Yoga Therapy Assessment (YTA) and the Anandamaya Kosha 209

3) Principles of Yoga Therapy Instruction (YTI) for the Anandamaya Kosha. 223

4) Purification of and Instruction for the Anandamaya Kosha 223

5) Prevention of Adverse Events in the Anandamaya Kosha. 233

6) Fictional Case Studies: Anandamaya Kosha 234

Part IV **Conclusion** 243

Chapter 1 Yoga Instruction and Adverse Events. 245

1) The Importance of Yoga Therapy Assessment (YTA) . . 245

2) Yoga Therapy Instruction (YTI) and Changes in the Client's Condition (CCC) 246

3) Conclusion. 247

About the Author. 249

Acknowledgments

First, I would like to express my gratitude to my guru, Swami Yogeshwarananda Maharaj. I had the great fortune and honor to study under him in the Himalayas during his last decade (from ages ninety to one hundred) and to receive direct transmission of all theory and practices in *Atma vijnana* (science of the soul), which use the five-sheath model of human structure. I have written about yoga therapy's theory and practice to address modern-day stress based on what I have learned from my guru.

I would also like to thank Dr. M. V. Bhole, professor emeritus of the Kaivalyadhama Yoga Research Institute, for his guidance in yoga therapy assessment, and Dr. H. R. Nagendra, president of the Swami Vivekananda Yoga Research Foundation, for his information on clinical practice. I also want to express my appreciation to all those at the Japan Yoga Therapy Society and Madoka Onizuka Chase who spent much time and effort to make publishing this book possible. Thank you very much.

Introduction

1) YOGA TODAY

I WENT TO INDIA FOR the first time in the 1970s as a college student eager to begin studying traditional yoga, and since then, I have dedicated myself to the practice, research, and promotion of yoga therapy. The world of yoga has changed dramatically over these past forty years.

When I first went to India, I was surprised to learn that yoga was not practiced as widely as I had expected. I met some curiosity seekers who tried their hands at asana, and some people practiced kundalini meditation to develop supernatural powers or fulfill materialistic and worldly goals. Then there were the yogis of the Himalayas, whose discipline was awe inspiring, and a few medical-college hospitals teaching yoga therapy and conducting yoga research.

Now, in the twenty-first century, it is estimated that some one hundred million people in India practice yoga asana and pranayama for the benefit of their health. This is a remarkable social phenomenon not limited to people from India. During my early visits, the only non-Indians I met who were practicing yoga seriously were either from the West or from Japan. Now, however, I see people from Russia, China, and other countries also going to India to study yoga. I believe this is due to the increased stress that economic development has brought to these newly industrialized nations.

This book introduces the key to overcoming stress. I provide both theoretical and practical information so that you can see how the traditional teachings of yoga can be adapted to the modern context and practiced by anyone. Yoga therapy not only addresses stress; it also contains the necessary theory and practice that enables us to transcend stress.

In 2003, I founded the Japan Yoga Therapy Society (JYTS) to promote yoga therapy in Japan, and to professionalize the field so that the quality of therapy is maintained and enhanced as our network and experience grows. JYTS started out as a small society, but it has grown rapidly. As of August 2016, we have 2,315 members, 1,453 of whom are certified yoga therapists. Our activities include yoga therapy instruction, instructor and therapist training courses, medical research in both Japan and the Ukraine, development of yoga therapy assessment tools, and contribution to international conferences in yoga therapy, psychosomatic medicine, and integrative medicine.

One of the studies JYTS conducted was entitled, "A large-scale survey of adverse events experienced in yoga classes,"[1] and it surveyed both students and teachers throughout Japan. It was done in cooperation with Dr. Takakazu Oka from the Department of Psychosomatic at the University of Kyushu's Graduate School of Medical Sciences and supported by the Ministry of Health, Labor and Welfare.

We surveyed 2,508 people attending regular yoga classes taught by yoga therapists in locations from Hokkaido to Okinawa, of mean age 58.5 ± 12.6 years (mean ± standard deviation). We also surveyed 271 yoga therapists. Class attendees were asked about adverse events[2] that they experienced, while yoga therapists were asked about adverse events that they observed in classes.

Of the class attendees, 1,343 (53.5 percent) reported having chronic illnesses, and 1,063 (42.3 percent) were receiving outpatient care at hospitals.

---

1 Tomoko Matsushita and Takakazu Oka, "A Large-Scale Survey of Adverse Events Experienced in Yoga Classes," *BioPsychoSocial Medicine* 9 (2015): 9.

2 An adverse event is, "any untoward medical occurrence that may arise during treatment with a pharmaceutical product but which does not necessarily have a causal relationship with this treatment." Source: http://medical-dictionary.thefreedictionary.com/adverse+event. Accessed Aug 22, 2016. The term is used here to refer to unpleasant or undesirable effects felt during yoga classes which may or may not have been due to a client's reaction to the yoga technique resulting from an already-existing medical condition.

Yoga Therapy Theory

This indicates that a significant number of people attending yoga classes have specific mental or physical disorders.

There is an international trend of people turning to yoga hoping for medical benefits, as evident in the changing yoga scene in both India and Japan. As both physical and mental stress intensifies with industrialization and a faster pace of life, we are seeing growing numbers of stress-related disorders. These disorders are also psychosomatic disorders, and many people are looking to yoga as a way to overcome them.

2) PURPOSE OF THIS BOOK

Yoga's physical practices have become immensely popular throughout the world in recent years, but traditional teachings that are at the foundation of the physical practices are less known. Even still, people are noticing the therapeutic effects of taking time to bring attention to one's own body and breath. In this book, I explain the ways traditional yoga looks at human structure and the functions fulfilled by various parts. Using specific verses from ancient scriptures, I will show how yoga's thousands of years of wisdom are relevant to the psychosomatic health issues we are facing today. Yoga therapy grounded in these teachings can work very well with conventional medical treatment to promote health in our societies. I also hope that increased understanding of traditional yogic teachings can help to address the dangerous trends I am noticing in the ways much modern yoga is taught. This book is based on a textbook used in the Japan Yoga Therapy Society's therapist training course, so it can be of practical use for yoga instructors and yoga therapists. It is my hope, however, that it will be of interest to anyone wanting to learn more about traditional yoga and its relevance to the health of our modern societies.

3) WHAT CAUSES ILLNESS?

Many medical advances have been made since the discovery of pathogens in the 1880s, and at one time, people thought that any disease could be

xiii

cured as long as the pathogen causing it could be identified and eradicated. We see today, however, that many diseases remain uncured in spite of the wide use of antibiotics, and there is no noticeable decline in the numbers of people visiting hospitals and clinics. This may be because we now have many illnesses different from those caused by bacteria and viruses. We have stress and lifestyle-related disorders that are both causing and being caused by the distress in our societies today.

As people become increasingly aware that unhealthy lifestyles lead to disease, it is no surprise that rather than depend on medical professionals, more people are looking for ways to cure themselves of the illnesses they themselves have created. They know that they need to take health back into their own hands to truly restore their health. It is also of no surprise to me that people are turning to a tradition that is thousands of years old and comes from the Himalayas. Yogis were not only able to endure incredible physical and mental stress while training in the Himalayas, they also lived happy and healthy lives there, thanks to the traditional yoga techniques they practiced. What better example could there be of a system to handle stress?

4) My First Encounters with Yoga Therapy

My first trip to India was in 1975, when the secrets of the yogis' mental and physical health were still not understood by the medical establishment. I initially went to the yoga university at the Kaivalyadhama Yoga Research Center in Maharashtra state, where physical changes brought about by yoga techniques were still being researched. Sometimes yogis would come to the research center next to the university to demonstrate rare techniques. Even if we were in the middle of class, we would stop what we were doing in order to go and watch. In this way, research was being conducted in the 1970s to understand the secrets of traditional yoga—and hence how to cope with stress. Such research is still under way today at universities and yoga research centers throughout India.

I was fortunate to be able to study the way I did. Thanks to the way in which things unfolded, I was able to audit courses, enabling me to sit in on all the classes without needing to take exams! Exempt from examinations, I took advantage of the long year-end holiday to go north to Rishikesh to Yoga Niketan, one of the traditional holy places to practice yoga. There, I met my life-long guru, Swami Yogeshwarananda Maharaj, who was ninety years old at the time. There were about two hundred people from both India and other countries, and from early in the morning until night, we practiced traditional Raja Yoga under my guru's instruction. I stayed for one month, during which I was able to receive instruction in Raja Yoga's asana, pranayama, and meditation directly from my guru.

That month at Yoga Niketan was so intense that even now, I am moved to tears of gratitude when I remember it. My guru was very generous in teaching us all the wisdom he attained in his many decades of Raja Yoga practice. The practices were teachings that had been handed down over many generations in the plateaus of the Himalayas and Tibet. Meditation methods and wisdom from the Vedas that had not reached Japan were transmitted to us disciples every day. Each day was like a duel of swords. We pushed our limits and challenged our guru in earnest, but our questions were often naïve or foolish. Still, there was always a sense of urgency in our efforts to attain real traditional wisdom. Every evening we had a two-hour *darshana*, a time in which we could ask our guru anything. It was also a time of counseling. I made sure to sit at my guru's feet every day without fail. Listening to his answers to the many and various questions, I tried to absorb the wisdom in his teachings.

After staying with my guru in Rishikesh for one month at the base of the Himalayas, I returned to the Kaivalyadhama Yoga Research Institute and attended college classes again. I remember early one Sunday morning I went to the second floor of the yoga hospital where there was a private room for foreign students. I started practicing the pranayama that I had learned from my guru. No one else was in the room, but upon hearing the severe sound of my breathing, a respected yoga therapist working at the hospital hurried into the room and told me to stop immediately. He reprimanded me, saying, "This is a yoga therapy facility. Don't show the patients the practices from the Himalayas." He explained that the pranayama I was practicing was traditional yoga and that patients should never be shown those techniques because they were too dangerous for them.

I was young and proud of having learned various traditional asana and pranayama practices. It was soon made clear to me, however, that traditional yoga practices were different from the yoga therapy techniques being studied at the research center. The college classes finished in March, and after that, I devoted myself to studying traditional Raja Yoga from the Himalayas under the guidance of my guru for ten years, until his death at age one hundred.

In 1987, as the turn of events would have it, I found it necessary to step into the field of yoga therapy. Now here I am, writing this book.

5) Theories of Human Structure and Function

In this book, I utilize vocabulary from conventional medicine and psychology to explain the yoga therapy methods used to correct defects in the mind-body complex. This refers specifically to (1) Yoga Therapy Assessment (YTA), (2) Yoga Therapy Instruction (YTI), and (3) yoga therapy practice, along with their theories and the mechanisms of how these three components of yoga therapy work to restore health.

In conventional medicine, doctors examine patients based on their knowledge of anatomy and physiology. Anatomy provides a definition of healthy human structure, and physiology provides a standard for healthy functions. Remember that these standards are being constantly revised as science develops. I am very concerned how, in contrast, many yoga instructors are teaching people with a diverse array of stress-related disorders without understanding yoga-based assessment or thinking sufficiently about traditional yoga's theory of instruction. To put it bluntly, there are many yoga instructors teaching asana and pranayama techniques that they themselves have often just learned. They are teaching these techniques before acquiring any real understanding of their effects. This makes their instruction haphazard and potentially dangerous.

The first step in yoga therapy is to assess where the mind-body system has broken down, and this assessment should be done based on traditional yogic teachings. Most yoga instructors, however, have neither the expertise nor theoretical understanding required to do this. There is a five-thousand-year tradition of yoga that has been handed down through generations of yogis in the Himalayas, and it provides very rigorous theory for assessment. This theory was essential to enable gurus to assess the mind-body conditions of their disciples in order to guide them to the highest stages of human character.

In traditional yoga, the theories of human structure (yoga's equivalent to anatomy) are the pancha kosha theory (five-sheath theory) from the *Taittiriya Upanishad*, and what I call the "human chariot theory" in the *Katha Upanishad*. The Upanishads are ancient scriptures said to be four thousand to five thousand years old.

Traditional yoga's "physiology" is found in the *Yoga Sutras* and other ancient scriptures. They explain how the functions of the mind-body complex can be disrupted, and yoga therapists can assess functional defects based on the teachings in the *Yoga Sutras*, the *Bhagavad Gita*, and other texts. While physiology addresses the body, yoga's "physiology" addresses the mind-body as one system. The teachings explain in depth about the human psyche and how it malfunctions.

Yoga therapy uses traditional yoga's theories of human structure and function to guide clients to the ideal state of being. Yoga therapists assess where there are malfunctions in their clients' bodies and minds, and it is possible to regulate and restore the functions to a healthy state.

In this book, I explain the pancha kosha and human chariot theories—yoga's "anatomy and physiology." I also explain methods to restore healthy human functions and the therapeutic effects of those methods, paying particular attention to techniques that can be used by people with various physical, mental, and psychosomatic disorders. Just as a medical doctor needs to understand the effects of medicines before prescribing them to patients, a yoga therapist must understand the effects of yoga therapy techniques before instructing their clients.

Yoga therapy instruction is not "treatment" in the sense of conventional medicine. Especially in the case of stress and lifestyle disorders, yoga therapy says that people create their own high blood pressure, ulcers, and psychological disorders. It is the role of yoga therapists to assist clients to become aware of the root causes of their own problems and to provide counseling and practices that empower clients to develop self-control and reclaim their health.

It is from this perspective that I explain traditional yoga practices and their effects, and how techniques have been adapted so that people who are vulnerable to stress and illness can practice them safely. For effective and safe practice of yoga, it is important that clients are assessed prior to beginning yoga therapy. Assessment should not be limited to the physical body, but should be done for physiological and psychological faculties as well.

Much of this book is dedicated to explaining the assessment theory we use at the Japan Yoga Therapy Society. It is based on the pancha kosha and human chariot theories that provide definitions of ideal human structure and standards to determine if the functioning of those structures is healthy. After assessment, programs are designed to help clients restore ideal human functions. This process is similar to what is done in conventional medicine. Finally, it is important to monitor clients' progress and the changes in their conditions, and evaluate whether or not clients are recovering ideal mental and physical conditions.

In addition to explaining the fundamental theory upon which yoga therapy assessment is based, I would also like to explain how yoga therapy should be instructed. This book has been written in simple terms to provide a basic understanding of the theories behind yoga therapy assessment and instruction, so if you are interested in more detail, please feel free to contact the Japan Yoga Therapy Society's head office.

6) Yoga Therapy and Ayurveda

A book on yoga therapy would not be complete without mentioning Ayurveda. Traditional yoga is a spiritual practice through which a practitioner can attain perfect health by becoming liberated from the ignorance that causes suffering. Traditional yoga, however, does not address medicines or what should be done when one falls ill with infectious or noncommunicable diseases. Ayurveda, on the other hand, is a medical science.

Yoga and Ayurveda are often spoken of as sister sciences, and they complement each other very well. While sharing very similar understandings of the human body and mind, yoga is focused on actual practices to guide healthy people to awaken to truth. Ayurveda helps restore balance that has been lost, using Ayurvedic medicines and other treatments. As you read further, it will become clearer how Ayurveda and yoga therapy can go hand in hand in promoting health.

The *Charaka Samhita* is one of the main texts used in Ayurveda, and it is said to have been compiled by the disciples of an Ayurvedic physician named Charaka who practiced around the first century. The *Charaka Samhita* explains three types of treatment—(1) rational, (2) spiritual, and (3) psychological. Of these, rational treatment is what is generally understood as medicine (i.e., using medicinal herbs and adjusting diet). The other two categories of Ayurveda are in the realm of yoga therapy. Yoga therapy covers mental and spiritual "treatment." In the *Charaka Samhita*, there are explanations of human structure and function that are actually almost the same as those found in the Upanishads, which I will explain in more detail in future chapters.

Charaka says that true health is achieved by total liberation from worldly matters, which is also addressed in traditional yoga. I explain in a little more detail about this as well. It can be said that Ayurveda and yoga share the same goal because both aim to guide us, as human beings, to the state of perfect health.

7) The Japan Yoga Therapy Society (JYTS)

Japan has a long history and has become a unique blend of East and West. Buddhism came to Japan about 1,500 years ago. Western medicine was introduced to Japan about 150 years ago. Japan was the first country in Asia to industrialize, and more scientists from Japan have been awarded Nobel Prizes than from any other Asian country.

The famous Swami Vivekananda also visited Japan on his way to the United States and strongly recommended the youth of India to visit Japan. I believe that our integration of East and West is why we at the Japan Yoga Therapy Society are successfully combining Western psychosomatic medicine with India's traditional yoga and Ayurveda to address modern stress-related and psychosomatic disorders. Having integrated the two, we have been able to develop our method of yoga therapy, which includes the components of Yoga Therapy Assessment (YTA), Yoga Therapy Instruction (YTI), and practice.

A. Instructor and Therapist Training

In Japan, we offer a Yoga Instructor Course (YIC) for people who want to learn how to teach yoga to healthy populations, and we have a Yoga Therapist Instructor Course (YTIC) for those who want to build on that knowledge to help clients with various mental and physical illnesses recover their health. Totaling 580 hours, our courses are offered in Japanese, but we are preparing to make them available in English. We also have ongoing education programs that certified yoga therapists are required to take to maintain certification (renewed every four years).

Our YIC is taught by Japan Yoga Niketan, which is registered with the Japanese Ministry of Education, Culture, Sports, Science, and Technology. The Japan Yoga Therapy Society is registered under the Japanese Ministry of Justice, and we are actively promoting yoga therapy, yoga therapy research, and academic activities. With this combination of traditional yoga and yoga therapy, we contribute to the recovery of health of many clients suffering from stress-related illnesses in Japan.

B. Annual Research Conference

Every year, we hold a research conference where two hundred to three hundred case studies are introduced in poster presentations. In addition, we invite medical professionals and researchers from around the world to speak at our conferences. Past speakers include Dr. Bessel van der Kolk, founder of the Trauma Center in Boston where yoga is being taught to help people overcome trauma, and Dr. Lorenzo Cohen of the MD Anderson Cancer Center and Director of the Center's Integrative Medicine Program. At our next conference in 2017, we are also looking forward to video conferencing with Dr. Herbert Benson, one of the pioneers in researching yoga from a medical perspective.

C. Research

The Japan Yoga Therapy Society is actively supporting and participating in research. We are developing yoga therapy assessment tools based on traditional scriptures, such as semi-structured interview manuals and questionnaires. We are also cooperating in research on yoga therapy for trauma, schizophrenia, gene expression, and dementia. We conducted the nation-wide study on adverse events in yoga mentioned earlier. Other examples of research we support are introduced in later parts of this book.

D. Volunteer Activities

Since 2011, the Japan Yoga Therapy Society has provided volunteer yoga therapy lessons for almost ten thousand people since the March 11 earthquake, tsunami, and nuclear disaster in northeastern Japan. In addition, we sent yoga therapists to Nepal after the earthquake in 2015 to teach yoga therapy to disaster victims and at evacuation sites just outside of Kathmandu. We taught approximately twelve hundred people over a three-month period.

We have also taught yoga therapy to people affected by the Chernobyl nuclear disaster, who are now living in Kiev. Since 2008, we have sent therapists once or twice a year to teach people who were exposed to radiation, and have provided training in how to teach yoga therapy to their local medical professionals and psychologists. We were inspired to begin this work because survivors of the bombings of Hiroshima and Nagasaki reported feeling benefits from practicing yoga therapy. Several survivors of the bombings have even graduated from our YTIC and are now teaching yoga therapy.

We also address the international problem of drug addiction, providing yoga therapy for people addicted to drugs in Japan as well as in Thailand. Since 2014, we have been providing yoga therapy education, including yoga therapy assessment, to the staff at the Princess Mother National Institute on Drug Abuse Treatment in Bangkok.

The content of this book is based on our achievements in all the preceding areas. Because this book is for the purposes of raising general awareness, I encourage people who would like to study in more detail to contact us. The isometric breathing exercises, isometric asana, and other techniques introduced in this book have been trademarked in Japan. We are applying for them to be trademarked in the United States as well. These are steps we are taking to ensure that our techniques are taught responsibly and safely. Because of the risk of adverse events, these exercises should not be taught without having completed the necessary training and having obtained permission from the Japan Yoga Therapy Society. Another indication of our growth as a professional organization is that yoga therapists certified by the Japan Yoga Therapy Society can now be covered by insurance for up to one hundred million yen (approximately 997,000 US dollars in 2016).

PART I

Yoga Therapy Theory: Theories of Human Structure and Function

CHAPTER 1

What is Yoga Therapy?

1) The Role of Yoga Therapists

Unlike traditional yoga practiced by ascetics in the Himalayas, yoga therapy has been developed for the public, be it people suffering from stress-related, lifestyle, and psychosomatic disorders, or people wanting to manage stress and prevent such illnesses.

In a cross-sectional study on adverse events and yoga that JYTS conducted and submitted to the Japan Ministry of Health and Welfare in 2013,[3] we surveyed 2,508 people attending yoga classes taught by yoga therapists certified by JYTS, and 1,343 (53.5 percent) of the respondents had some type of chronic ailment. From what I have observed in Japan, many people with health problems of varying degrees of severity go to yoga classes looking for some kind of relief or health benefits, whether or not the classes are taught by yoga therapists. I see this happening in other countries as well.

Considering the numbers of people looking to yoga for health benefits, it is important that yoga therapists, yoga instructors, and their clients understand that yoga therapy is not traditional yoga. By "traditional yoga," I am referring to yoga that has been passed down over thousands of years in the Himalayas for the purpose of spiritual enlightenment. Yoga therapy adapts the physically and mentally challenging practices of traditional yoga so that they can be practiced to benefit people living in

---

3 Matsushita and Oka, "A Large-Scale Survey of Adverse Events Experienced in Yoga Classes, 9 (doi 10. 1186/s 13030-015-0037-1).

high-stress urban environments. What is it that needs to be taught in this social context?

Remember that there are people coming to yoga classes wanting to address illnesses or prevent disease. It is, therefore, necessary to assess students' conditions *prior to* instruction of yoga techniques. In 2011, M. V. Bhole, a doctor and professor at the Kaivalyadhama Yoga Institute, came to Tokyo to conduct a yoga therapy seminar. In this seminar, he explained the need for assessing and monitoring clients as follows:

> Yoga therapists must first conduct a yoga therapy assessment, which is an intake of first-time students or clients. Based on this assessment, the client's condition should be understood, and an evaluation made regarding the expected changes in symptoms, so that it can be decided what practices should be used in yoga therapy to guide clients back to restored health. Upon explaining the yoga therapy plan, the changes that the client can expect to feel, and the expected outcomes of the practice, therapists should obtain the client's informed consent to practice the program.

The first step in yoga therapy is for the yoga therapist to assess a client's mental and physical condition with an intake interview, design a program based on the assessment, and obtain the consent of the client. The unfortunate reality is that instead, an instructor might simply say, "Yoga is good for you. We'll all practice together, but if something doesn't feel right, don't push yourself too far and feel free to stop."

It is important for clients to know that they can stop, but beginners often do not know how far is "too far." They do not know how things are supposed to feel, so they might not have confidence to say something does not feel right. Such vague instruction is bound to lead to adverse events, much less promote health. To prevent accidents, yoga therapists should not rely on these vague statements, but must make sure to assess first-time clients to ensure that they do not tell the clients to practice techniques that are unsuitable for their condition.

Yoga Therapy Theory

In general yoga classes or in yoga therapy, it is impossible to teach asana, pranayama, and meditation according to the needs of the individual without knowing if a new student is hoping to overcome panic attacks, prevent recurrence of cancer, or is taking leave from work due to depression. This should be common sense. It is no different from a medical doctor prescribing medicine without conducting an initial examination or making a diagnosis. Yoga instructors also need to have a clear understanding of the physiological and psychological effects of yoga techniques as therapy, or else their teaching cannot help but be vague.

Yoga teachers sometimes claim that a specific pose is good for a specific illness, but there is no medical research to support such claims. One pose is not going to cure an illness, but instructors make such claims without evidence to back up their statements. This happens not only in Japan, but also in yoga classes around the world. This misunderstanding of yoga is not only misinformed, but is potentially dangerous and can lead to serious adverse events. One of the reasons I am writing this book is to contribute to developing a more holistic understanding of yoga among those who are teaching, and to develop a safer system of instruction.

For the preceding reason, this book is primarily for people already teaching yoga, but I also hope it is a useful reference for people struggling with various ailments. Some yoga therapy techniques are introduced later in this book, and they can be practiced at home. To practice more advanced yoga therapy techniques that are appropriate for your mental and physical condition, it is important to study under the instruction of a qualified yoga therapist.

2) The Difference Between Yoga Instructors and Yoga Therapists

In addition to emphasizing the need for better yoga therapy assessments, Dr. Bhole explained the difference between yoga and yoga therapy. As I mentioned earlier, Dr. Bhole worked at the Kaivalyadhama Yoga Institute, which was founded in the 1920s and led the world in scientific research on traditional yoga at the time. Dr. Bhole worked there for thirty years and has played an important role in informing the world about yoga therapy. We were fortunate to have him lecture in Japan twice between 2008 and 2011. During his lectures, he explained yoga therapy and the difference between yoga therapists and yoga instructors as follows.

What is yoga therapy? It is one of the most appropriate methods for managing stress to overcome illness and maintain health, and it can be incorporated into one's lifestyle. It can also enable you to experience samadhi, or complete physical and mental integration. And what are the characteristics of yoga therapy? There are many types of medical treatments in conventional medicine, but the patient is passive in all of them. Sometimes they are even put to sleep with anesthesia. However, under the instruction of a yoga therapist, a patient learns ways to improve their own health and practice those techniques on their own. Unlike other treatment modalities, patients are actively involved in healing themselves.

What is the difference between a yoga instructor and a yoga therapist? Yoga instructors are usually technique oriented in their training, thinking and oral approach. In medical terms, they could be looked upon as yoga pharmacists. Yoga therapists, on the other hand, are expected to be individual oriented in their training, thinking and approach. In medical terms, they have to become yoga physicians. Therefore, apart from the details of different yoga techniques, yoga therapists should also be equipped with the following: the knowledge about the organization of normal human consciousness and how it gets disturbed, and how to help an individual return to the normal state of consciousness, if or when disturbed. Various yoga practices could be looked upon as yogic intervention techniques, very much similar to drugs, surgical and/or psychological procedures. One of the present deficiencies or shortcomings of yoga therapy is that there are no standardized methods of establishing yogic diagnosis. Diagnoses done by specialists of other treatment modalities are generally used for yoga therapy. There is no yogic pharmacopeia or yogic *materia medica* today. It needs to be developed. The present research in the field of yoga therapy is directed to the treatment of specific diseases such as diabetes, asthma, heart conditions etc. We want evidence-based knowledge in respect to different yoga techniques. From the perspective of yoga therapy, health problems can be divided into two categories. One is the medical/surgical category, where medical treatment is primary and yoga is secondary. The other is the psycho-spiritual category, where yoga treatment is primary and medical treatment is secondary.

Dr. Bhole's words carry great weight as an experienced medical doctor having dedicated much of his life to yoga therapy research at the Kaivalyadhama Yoga Research Institute. I realized the importance of his analysis of the challenges facing yoga therapy as a field. It inspired me to begin working with doctors and psychologists in Japan to develop methods and diagnostic tools for yoga-based assessments of mental and physical health, and I explain these and the theory behind them in this book. I hope that this book will contribute to the body of knowledge of yoga therapy and help people better understand the medical and psychological effects of yoga.

3) Ayurveda: India's Traditional Medicine

Ayurveda is said to have its roots in the *Atharva Veda*, one part of the Vedas, holy scriptures from ancient India. Charaka was a great physician who taught extensively on Ayurveda. He traveled throughout India and taught his disciples many methods of medical treatment, and his disciples compiled his teachings into a medical text that is now known as the *Charaka Samhita*. Currently more than two hundred medical departments in universities in India offer Ayurveda courses alongside conventional medicine. Similar to doctors of conventional medicine, to qualify as an Ayurvedic doctor requires five and a half years of medical education and research in Ayurveda. Though written two thousand years ago, the *Charaka Samhita* is still a very important text taught in medical colleges and used in clinical settings even today. Volume I, chapter 11.54 contains an explanation of types of therapy.

Charaka Samhita Sutra Sthana **Chapter 11, Verse 54**[4]

Therapies are of three kinds, viz., spiritual therapy, therapy based on reasoning (physical propriety) and psychic therapy. Spiritual therapies are incantation of mantras, talisman, wearing of gems, auspicious offering, gifts, oblations, observance of scriptural rules, atonement, fasts, chanting of auspicious hymns, obeisance to the gods, going on pilgrimage, etc., administration of proper diet and medicinal drugs comes under the second category. Withdrawal of mind from harmful objects constitutes psychic therapy.

Commentary

In Japan, Ayurveda is generally thought of as oil massage for beauty and relaxation. Particularly well known are *abhyanga* and *shirodhara*, which are treatments involving massage and pouring herbal oil on the forehead. These are only two of a vast array of treatments, however, and they belong to the category of rational therapy. Charaka explains that there are two additional categories in Ayurveda—spiritual therapy and psychological therapy. These two categories examine the mind-body relationship in disease and

---

4 All references from the *Charaka Samhita* come from *Agnivesa's Caraka Samhita, Text with English Translation and Critical Exposition Based on (Cakrapani Datta's Ayurveda Dipika)*, by Ram Karan Sharma and Vaidya Bhagwan Dash, (Varanasi, India: Chowkhamba Sanskrit Series Office, 2015), 231.
Note: In the original source texts, including this one and others, Sanskrit words are written using diacritic marks that indicate pronunciation that cannot be expressed with the English alphabet. Due to inability to use diacritic marks in this book, spelling of Sanskrit words has been changed to the closest English equivalent.

health, and are areas directly addressed by yoga therapy. These words by Charaka make it clear that yoga and Ayurveda are sister sciences.

Also interesting to note is that pathology at the time of Charaka did not involve pathogens as the causes of disease. Charaka explains pathology in the following verse.

Charaka Samhita Vimanasthana Chapter 6 Verse 5[5]

Because of their highly multitudinous nature, diseases are innumerable. On the other hand, doshas are numerable because of their limitation in number. So only some of the diseases will be explained by way of illustrations whereas doshas will be explained in their entirety. Rajas *and* tamas *are the doshas pertaining to the mind and the types of morbidity caused by them are kama (passion), anger, greed, attachment, envy, ego, pride, grief, worry, anxiety, fear, excitement etc.* Vata, pitta, *and* kapha— *these three are the doshas pertaining to the body. Diseases caused by them are fever, diarrhoea, oedema, consumption, dyspnea,* meha *(obstinate urinary disorder including diabetes),* kustha *(obstinate skin diseases including leprosy) etc. Thus doshas in their entirety and diseases in parts are explained.*

Commentary

We all know that if we are mentally and physically strong and have sufficient immunity, exposure to pathogens will not necessarily make us sick. We also know that antibiotics are of no use for stress-related disorders that arise regardless of bacteria and viruses. In Ayurveda, the cause of human disease is said to be due to doshas.

---

5 *Caraka Samhita* vol. II, 186.

There are two types of doshas (vitiating factors that cause disease), physical and psychological, and Charaka explains their relationship in the following verse.

Charaka Samhita Vimanasthana Chapter 6 Verse 8[6]

When allowed to persist for long, these psychic diseases, viz., kama (passion) etc., and somatic diseases viz., fever etc., at times get combined with each other.

Commentary

Charaka's explanation of pathogenesis attributes disease to a disruption in the relationship between mind and body, which then leads to various diseases manifesting in the physical body. In the 1800s, when bacteria were discovered, this way of thinking fell away; however, as societies have industrialized and become increasingly stressful, we are seeing a proliferation of stress-related illnesses around the world as the balance between mind and body breaks down. With this we are also seeing the Ayurvedic and yogic ways of thinking being reconsidered and revived. Charaka places great importance on the relationship between mind and body, and makes it clear that Ayurveda and yoga contain the wisdom needed to assess human disorders and restore both mental and physical health. Moreover, Charaka says that it is the mental disturbances in the mind-body relationship that are the root causes of disease.

Charaka Samhita Sharira Sthana Chapter 4 Verse 34[7]

Now, there are three physical doshas *(vitiating elements), viz.,* vata, pitta, *and* kapha—*they vitiate the body. Again there are two mental* doshas, *viz.,* rajas, *and* tamas—*they vitiate the mind. Vitiation of the body and*

---

6 *Caraka Samhita* vol. II, 187.
7 *Caraka Samhita* vol. II, 405.

the mind result in the manifestation of diseases—there is no disease without their vitiation.

Commentary

In this verse, Charaka explains that diseases of the body are caused by physical doshas. Doshas are elements that bring about a specific type of change. Diseases of the mind are caused by mental doshas. Illness results when the effects of these doshas create imbalance in the mind and/or body.

Charaka goes on to explains mental disturbances as follows:

Charaka Samhita: Sharira Sthana **Chapter 4 Verse 36**[8]

Mental faculty is of three types—sattvika, rajasa and tamasa. The sattvika one is free from defects as it is endowed with auspiciousness. The rajas type is defective because it promotes wrathful disposition. The tamasa one is similarly defective because it suffers from ignorance.

Each of the three types of mental faculty is in fact of innumerable variety by permutation and combination of the various factors relating to the body, species and mutual interactions. Sometimes even the body follows the mind and vice versa. So we shall now explain some of the varieties of mental faculties briefly by way of illustration.

Commentary

In this verse, Charaka makes it clear that the mental and physical doshas affect each other, and the disruptions in the mind affect the body and vice versa. This understanding of mind-body interactions is also found in modern psychosomatic medicine. To explain in more detail, changes are constantly occurring in the

---

8 *Caraka Samhita* vol. II, 406.

human psyche. The psyche is controlled by three gunas, namely sattva, rajas, and tamas. At any point in time, one of these gunas is predominant, and the predominant one determines the state of a person's mind at that time. Of the three gunas, rajas, and tamas are also called doshas (because they are vitiating), and when imbalanced, they are said to be responsible for disease. Rajas and tamas never disappear completely, but can take an inferior position to sattva. If we want to live a mentally and physically healthy life, then effort is needed to keep the sattva guna as predominant as possible. Predominance of sattva guna in our mental condition is also part of promoting the health of our physical body. This is where yoga therapy comes in. It has many techniques to help people develop more self-control and sattvic conditions, promoting the health of people living in modern, stressful societies. This is why instructors of yoga in this modern age need to study and understand the psychology of traditional yoga.

I hope it is clear that yoga therapy is significant as a practice that covers two of Ayurveda's types of treatments, that is, psychological and spiritual therapy.

Yoga therapy addresses psychosomatic disorders and lifestyle diseases that are not the result of bacteria or other pathogens. It is a mind-body practice that helps people manage the stresses of modern society which are leading to many psychosomatic disorders. The theory of diagnosis and treatment in Ayurveda is the foundation for yoga therapy assessment and instruction. This will become clearer in the following section, where I will explain more about yoga therapy techniques.

4) Three Categories of Yoga Therapy Techniques

Traditional yoga can be divided largely into the four schools of Jnana Yoga, Bhakti Yoga, Karma Yoga, and Raja Yoga. The fourth, Raja Yoga, includes techniques from all the schools, and hence its name. "Raja" means "king," making Raja Yoga the "king of yoga." It is a comprehensive path.

Yoga Therapy Theory

Modern yoga therapy bases itself on Raja Yoga to promote health. Of the Raja Yoga practices used in yoga therapy, the most common are asana, pranayama (breathing exercises), and meditation.

Asana: Physical Practice

In traditional yoga, asanas make up much of the physical practice. "Asana" literally means, "posture for sitting in meditation." The main purpose of asana practice is to cultivate the physical body so that it can tolerate sitting in meditation for super-human lengths of time. My guru used to enter samadhi while sitting in a meditation posture not just for several hours, but sometimes for more than ten days without eating or drinking. There are several hundred asanas, and they are for cultivating the strength of both body and mind for meditation. Yogis also developed techniques that they needed to cultivate strength to walk thousands of kilometers in the Himalayas, to climb steep cliffs with their bare hands, to cross rivers without bridges, and to stay warm while crossing glaciers without the modern equipment we have today.

Yoga therapists certified by the Japan Yoga Therapy Society teach easy isometric asanas as yoga therapy. Isometric asanas retain the essence of these traditional yoga practices and enable elderly and people with health problems to practice them safely. In Japan, these asana practices are promoting health, enabling elderly people to live independently, and people with stress-related illnesses are recovering and reclaiming their health. In part III of this book, I will introduce some case studies that illustrate the effects we are seeing with yoga therapy in Japan. For now, let me explain the two classifications of strength training that we use in our asana instruction—isometric and isotonic training.

Speaking in exercise physiology terms, there are isometric and isotonic muscle contractions, and my guru and his disciples used both. Yoga therapy retains the essence of traditional yoga asana strength training, but the methods are adapted so that anyone can benefit from the practices that build both physical and psychological strength, train the brain, balance the autonomic nervous system, and promote the functions of the immune system. These medical and psychological benefits are being proven by a growing body of scientific research on yoga and yoga therapy being conducted around the world.

PRANAYAMA: BREATHING TECHNIQUES

There are many pranayama practices in traditional yoga. When I was studying in the Himalayas with my guru, I learned more than one hundred pranayama practices directly from him. My guru also learned those same practices from his guru, Holy Guru Paramananda Avaduta, when he went as a teenager to the western part of the Himalayas to an area called Sonamarg in the mountains of Kashmir. Guru Paramananda Avaduta also learned those practices from his guru, Holy Guru Atmananda in western Tibet near Mount Kailash, in a sacred area called Tirthapuri. In this way, the pranayama practices passed down over generations in the Himalayas are of a completely different level than the practices generally taught in yoga classes today. Opportunities to receive these traditional teaching are given only to those who can prove the passion and determination to learn.

When teaching people for the promotion of health, we cannot teach the same traditional pranayama techniques that have been handed down in the Himalayas. Clients do not have the physical and mental strength of yogis in the Himalayas, so to try such practices would immediately lead to adverse events. In my own forty years of yoga practice, I have seen several people suffer damaging effects of certain pranayama practices. Without understanding the traditional teachings nor the difference between traditional yoga and yoga therapy, and neglecting to follow the instructions of their guru, they assumed more repetitions would bring more benefit. They did too much, and it had terrible consequences on their health. The breathing exercises introduced in this book have been adapted in order to avoid and prevent such adverse events.

As one yoga-therapy technique, JYTS developed breathing exercises that combine asana and pranayama into one practice. In particular, we developed a technique that we call, "isometric breathing exercise," which incorporates the essence of traditional yoga practices done by yogis in the Himalayas that strengthen both body and mind. This technique has been registered and trademarked under the patent office as a technique developed by the JTYS. If you are interested in practicing these techniques, make sure that you receive instruction from a yoga therapist certified by the Japan Yoga Therapy Society.

VEDIC MEDITATION: YOGA PSYCHOTHERAPY

Meditation techniques practiced in traditional yoga are explained in the Upanishads. When I practiced meditation with my guru in the Himalayas, he guided his disciples according to the four stages explained subsequently. This method was developed before the birth of the Buddha, and one practice explained in the *Brihadaranyaka Upanishad*, famous among the ancient Upanishads, is what we now call vedic meditation. In chapter II verse 4.5, there is a famous conversation between Yajnavalkya and his wife, Maitreyi, in which Yajnavalkya explains the steps of meditation.

Brihadaranyaka Upanishad Chapter II Verse 4.5[9]

A wife loves her husband not for his own sake, dear, but because the Self lives in him.

A husband loves his wife not for her own sake, dear, but because the Self lives in her.

...Everything is loved not for its own sake, but because the Self lives in it.

This Self has to be realized. Hear about this Self and meditate upon him, Maitreyi. When you hear about the Self, meditate upon the Self, and finally realize the Self, you come to understand everything in life.

---

9 All *Upanishad* references come from the translation by Eknath Easwaran. Eknath Easwaran, *The Upanishads*. Introduction and translation. (Nilgiri Press, Tomales, Canada, 2009), 100 (hereafter cited as *The Upanishads*).

Commentary

In this verse, Yajnavalkya is explaining the sadhana (practice) to reach ultimate liberation after being asked to do so by his wife, Maytreyi. He explains the four stages of meditation. In the first stage called *shravana*, one listens carefully to a teacher and studies the sacred texts. This is the stage of the Self being heard. In the second stage, one contemplates the teachings. It is a stage of reflection called *manana*. The third stage is *nididhyasana*, in which one integrates the contemplation into one's daily life, and this is very deep meditation. After this, it is said that one can reach the last stage called *jnana*, or the realization of one's own true nature, that is to know the Self.

These fundamental meditation techniques are also introduced in the first chapter of *Panchadashi*, a text written in the late fourteenth century by Swami Vidyaranya, who held the position of Shankaracharya at the Shringeri Monastery in southern India from 1377 to 1386.

Panchadashi[10] Verse 1–53

The finding out or discovery of the true significance of the identity of the individual self and the Supreme with the aid of the great sayings (like Tattvamasi) is what is known as shravana. And to arrive at the possibility of its validity thorough logical reasoning is what is called manana.

Panchadashi Verse 1–54

And, when by shravana and manana the mind develops a firm and undoubted conviction, and dwells constantly on the thus ascertained Self alone, it is called unbroken meditation (nididhyasana).

---

10 All excerpts from *Panchadashi* are from Vidyaranya Swami, *Panchadasi*, trans. Swami Swahananda (Chennai, India: Sri Ramakrishna Math). Accessed August 1, 2016, http://www.celextel.org/othervedantabooks/panchadasi.html.

Panchadashi Verse 1–55

When the mind gradually leaves off the ideas of the meditator and the act of meditation and is merged in the sole object of meditation (viz., the Self), and is steady like the flame of a lamp in a breezeless spot, it is called the superconscious state (samadhi).

Commentary

Unfortunately, these traditional techniques introduced in the Vedas are not widely known in Japan, so even though many people speak about meditation, skilled and precise instruction of traditional meditation is not common. This Vedic meditation is a particularly effective yoga therapy tool that helps clients who are full of worldly passions to notice, reevaluate, and correct their mistaken cognition that causes them stress and suffering. I will introduce some techniques in this book.

The job of the yoga therapist is to combine the preceding three techniques of asana, pranayama, and meditation in a way that is best suited to facilitate the client's return to a healthy mental and physical condition.

In the next chapter, I will briefly explain the theory of human structure as taught in traditional yoga, which is very important to understand for yoga therapy instruction. Its role in yoga therapy is similar to the role that anatomy plays in conventional medicine.

CHAPTER 2

Yoga's Theory of Human Structure and its

Application to Stress Management

VARIOUS MEDICAL SCIENCES AND MODALITIES have different standards defining healthy human condition. In conventional medicine, for example, anatomy and physiology define the healthy structure and functions of the human body. A person's physical condition is compared to what has been defined as healthy, and if there are differences, problems are diagnosed, and then treatment is chosen with the goal of returning the person to a healthy state, as defined by anatomy and physiology.

Another modality that has gained international recognition is Chinese medicine, and it uses theories of yin-yang and the five elements to explain human function and structure, theories different from the anatomy and physiology used in conventional medicine. Using these theories, Chinese medicine distinguishes between what is normal and defective functioning, and has its own methods for restoring health.

In India, traditional yoga also has theories of human structure and function, which I will introduce in this chapter. When these structures or functions break down and illnesses occur, Ayurveda's three categories of treatment are used to restore a person to a healthy condition. One of the three categories in Ayurveda is rational treatment, in which specific diet and medicines are prescribed. The other two categories of psychological and spiritual treatments are addressed by yoga therapy, as explained in section 3 of the previous chapter.

To use yoga for education and therapy, it is necessary to understand how yoga looks at human structure and function. These teachings have been handed down for more than four thousand years and are still relevant today. I will explain in more detail subsequently, introducing references from ancient texts.

1) THE THEORY OF HUMAN STRUCTURE AS WRITTEN IN THE TAITTIRIYA UPANISHAD (PANCHA KOSHA THEORY)

In ancient India, human structure was explained as five sheaths, known as pancha kosha. This is explained in the Upanishads, particularly in the *Taittiriya Upanishad*, which was written sometime between 3000 and 2000 BC. The explanation is given in a conversation between a father and his son.

Taittiriya Upanishad Part III 1.1[11]

> *Bhrigu went to his father, Varuna,*
> *and asked respectfully: "What is Brahman?"*
> *Varuna replied: "First learn about food,*
> *Breath, eye, ear, speech, and mind; then seek to know*
> *That from which these are born, by which they live,*
> *For which they search, and to which they return.*
> *That is Brahman."*

Commentary

Bhrigu asks his father about Brahman, that is, the source of everything temporal, the Universal Self. Varuna is wise and knows that his son must meditate to really understand. He therefore tells Bhrigu to meditate first on food and continues to guide him through subsequent verses to finally come the realization of "that

---

11 *The Upanishads*, 257.

from which everything is born and to which everything returns." In traditional yoga, we are taught that relying on things in the ever-changing material world creates suffering, and that it is better to find stability from that which is immovable and does not change.

It is evident that psychosomatic and lifestyle diseases are emerging from the stresses created by overreliance on worldly things that change. In Japan, we have an expression that the three main stressors leading to illness are human relationships, money, and pride. All of these are changeable, and yet people often cling to them in hope of finding security. By understanding the pancha kosha theory, we can understand how to lead a healthy life. It contains the answer to guide us out of seeking identity and security in the temporal. Instead, we learn to unite with that which is immoveable, immortal, and indestructible.

After Bhrigu meditates on food, he was not satisfied, and goes to his father asking for more instruction.

Taittiriya Upanishad Part III 2.1[12]

> *Bhrigu meditated and found that food*
> *Is Brahman. From food are born all creatures,*
> *By food they grow, and to food they return.*
> *Not fully satisfied with his knowledge,*
> *Bhrigu went to his father, Varuna,*
> *And appealed; "Please teach me more of Brahman."*
> *"Seek it through meditation," replied Varuna,*
> *"For meditation is Brahman."*

---

12 *The Upanishads*, 257.

Commentary

From this verse in the *Taittiriya Upanishad* onward, Varuna and his son, Bhrigu, discuss the five koshas.

While I studied with my guru Swami Yogeshwarananda Maharaj in the Himalayas, we trained every day in *Atma vijnana*, or "science of the soul," in order to realize our true Self (*Atman*). This understanding of the five koshas has been the foundation of practice to realize *Atman* for over five thousand years. The theory behind this discipline is the pancha kosha theory itself. In other words, our daily discipline enabled us to see these koshas objectively and come to the unshakable realization that the five sheaths, beginning with the food sheath or physical body, are not the true Self.

At the time, my guru was ninety years old, and he had been practicing for eighty years. He explained to us that he was initiated into this practice of *Atma vijnana* by Mahatma Atmananda Maharaj, who is said to have lived for more than three hundred years in the sacred region of Tirthapuri in Tibet. Indeed, the description in the preceding verse of the *Taittiriya Upanishad* is precisely what I learned in the Vedic meditation I practiced with my Guru every day in the Himalayas.

Varuna and Bhrigu continue to discuss the five sheaths of human existence—the annamaya kosha (physical sheath), pranamaya kosha (vital air sheath), manomaya kosha (mind sheath, composed of the organs of perception and action), vijnanamaya kosha (intellect sheath), and the anandamaya kosha (bliss sheath). Through contemplation and meditation, Bhrigu comes to the understanding that these five koshas are not the real Self. He realizes *Atman*, the real Self, the innermost entity that is the individualized manifestation of the universal Brahman.

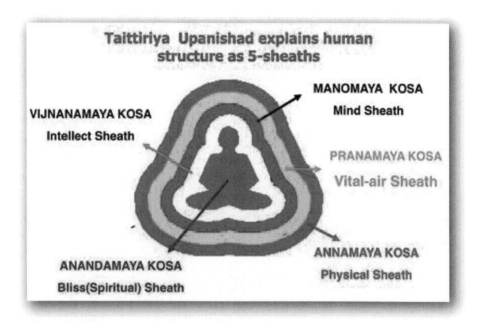

Figure 1. An illustration of the pancha kosha. The pancha kosha theory enables us to understand the human system as five layers—the annamaya, pranamaya, manomaya, vijnanamaya, and anandamaya koshas—and assess the defects in their functions and what needs to be done to return them to a healthy condition. I will write a more detailed explanation of each kosha in section 3 of this chapter.

I will now introduce the verse that explains the anandamaya kosha, the innermost of the five koshas.

Taittiriya Upanishad **Part III 6.1**[13]

> *Bhrigu meditated and found that joy*
> *Is Brahman. From joy are born all creatures,*
> *By joy they grow, and to joy they return.*
> *Bhrigu, Varuna's son, realized this Self*
> *In the very depths of meditation.*

---

13 *The Upanishads*, 258.

Those who realize the Self within the heart
Stand firm, grow rich, gather a family
Around them, and receive the love of all.

Commentary

The discussion between Varuna and Bhrigu concludes with the anandamaya kosha (bliss sheath), but this Upanishad does not say that this last kosha is the equivalent of Atman. The anandamaya kosha is the fifth kosha, and even deeper within is the real Self, *Atman*, the force that gives birth to all koshas. It contains two of four psychological organs—the ahamkara and chitta. Sages from ancient times have said that the chitta is the storehouse of all memory.

The *Yoga Sutras*, compiled by Patanjali around 300 BC and considered to be one of the authoritative texts on Raja Yoga, defines memory in verse 1.11 as:
Memory is not allowing an object which has been experienced to escape.

In Verse 1. 2, Patanjali defines yoga as the suppression of the modifications of the chitta, the storehouse of memory. So what Patanjali is saying here is that the aim of yoga is to suppress all the activities of old memories, including memories that have been forgotten but that are still stored in the chitta. These various kinds of memories, including trauma and posttraumatic stress disorder (PTSD), can inflict great suffering. Upon freeing oneself from the mistaken identification with this storehouse of memory, one arrives at the final true Self/*Atman*, the ultimate goal.

Conventional medicine only addresses health of the outermost sheath, the "food sheath," or the annamaya kosha. This is not sufficient to maintain or restore health of the whole person, and this is why we are seeing more specialists in conventional medicine showing interest in the mind-body connection in psychosomatic medicine. We yoga therapists are able to work together with these specialists to help promote the health of patients because yoga therapy addresses both body and mind. Yoga therapy also derives its techniques from practices that have been developed over thousands of years. In a manner of speaking, generations of yogis have experimented on themselves and proven the effects of these methods to control body and mind.

2) The *Katha Upanishad* "Human Chariot Theory"

There is one more theory that explains human structure, and it is written in the *Katha Upanishad*. There is only one reason for the emergence of these theories of what comprises a human being, including the pancha kosha theory. The yogis from long ago wanted to know how to skillfully control this constantly changing body and mind. Just as in the case of an airplane or car, if one does not know the structure and functions of the parts, one cannot maneuver it well, and there is a danger of mishandling. It is clear that the pancha kosha theory and chariot metaphor that I will explain next are very useful for understanding the structure and functions of the human system. If they were not useful, they would not have been handed down for five thousand years. Allow me now to introduce the chariot metaphor, or what I call the "human chariot theory" from chapter III of the *Katha Upanishad*.

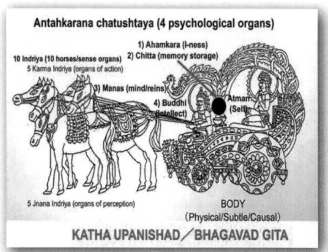

Figure 2. The human chariot model from the *Katha Upanishad*.

The human chariot theory appears in chapter III of the *Katha Upanishad* in a conversation between a pure young prince named Nachiketa and Yama, the lord of death. The prince is sent away by his angry father to Lord Yama as punishment, but Yama is not there when he arrives. Nachiketa waits for three days and three nights for Yama to return.

When Yama returns, he is impressed by Nachiketa's forbearance and promises to fulfill three wishes, no matter what they may be. Nachiketa first asks to be reconciled with his father. Second, he asks to know how to conduct the fire ceremony to go to heaven. Yama, the lord of death, grants these two wishes. Then Nachiketa asks for his third in the following verse.

Katha Upanishad **Chapter III Part I Verse 1.20**[14]

When a person dies, there arises this doubt: "He still exists," say some; "he does not," say others. I want you to teach me the truth. This is my third boon.

Commentary

For his third wish, Nachiketa asks Yama to teach him the secret of death and eternity. This alarms Yama, who does not want to disclose the knowledge of how to transcend heaven and hell. This is the wisdom that successive yogis have sought to discover since ancient times; to attain the wisdom of Brahman. Those who realize Brahman can slip through the fingers of Yama.

Yama tries in vein to tempt Nachiketa with wealth, long life, and prosperity for his descendants. Nachiketa knows these things are limited and rejects them all. He insists that he wants to know that which is absolute. Yama gives in, and it is in chapter 3 of the *Katha Upanishad* that Yama reveals to Nachiketa the answer to his third question. To reach absolute truth, understand and conduct oneself in accordance with the human chariot model, which Yama begins to explain in the following verse.

---

14 *The Upanishads*, 72.

Katha Upanishad **Chapter III Part I Verse 3.3**[15]

> *Know the Self as lord of the Chariot,*
> *The body as the chariot itself,*
> *The discriminating intellect as*
> *The charioteer, and the mind as reins.*

Yama continues his explanation, describing the horses drawing the chariot as the senses and their relationship to the reins and driver.

Katha Upanishad **Chapter III Part I Verse 3.4**[16]

> *The senses, say the wise, are the horses;*
> *Selfish desires are the roads they travel.*
> *When the Self is confused with the body,*
> *Mind, and the senses, they point out, he seems*
> *To enjoy pleasure and suffer sorrow.*

Commentary

Ordinarily, people want to obtain the objects of the senses, or things that bring pleasure. When people identify themselves with the body, senses, and mind, obtaining objects becomes important because without them, they feel incomplete. When this mistaken identification is too strong, people succumb to various lifestyle diseases, psychosomatic diseases, and psychological disorders.

---

15 *The Upanishads*, 81.
16 *The Upanishads*, 81.

Katha Upanishad Chapter III Part I Verse 3.5[17]

When a person lacks discrimination
And his mind is undisciplined, the senses
Run hither and thither like wild horses.

Commentary

This is one example of how we can use the Katha Upanishads to assess personality traits, such as attachment to sensory objects to find fulfillment. That is to say, if the mental and physical functions of a person are as uncontrollable as ten wild horses that do not heed the reins of a chariot driver, life will be dangerous, like a runaway chariot at the mercy of desire for sensory satisfaction.

Katha Upanishad Chapter III Part I Verse 3.6[18]

But they obey the rein like trained horses
When one has discrimination and
Has made the mind one-pointed.

Commentary

This verse explains that if the buddhi (intellect/charioteer) is wise, it makes sound decisions and can rein in the horses. It can recognize the reality of a situation, so even if the ten horses are overreacting to events of the outside world, the buddhi can skillfully control them. In everyday life, and even in times of great stress, there will be no addiction or overreliance on harmful pleasures. This is what is explained in this yogic "functional theory" of the human mind-body complex.

---

17 *The Upanishads*, 81.
18 *The Upanishads*, 81.

Katha Upanishad Chapter III Part I Verse 3.7[19]

Those who lack
Discrimination, with little control
Over their thoughts and far from pure,
Reach not the pure state of immortality
But wander from death to death;

Commentary

Regardless of whether or not one believes in reincarnation, living for decades unable to control the rowdy horses (organs of perception and action) will disrupt mental balance and affect not only the central nervous system, but also the endocrine system and immune system. Physical organs in the body will also certainly be affected. This has the potential to make life miserable. So regardless of the issue of rebirth, it is clear that the quality of this life itself is at risk if psychosomatic and lifestyle disorders are prominent.

Katha Upanishad Chapter III Part I Verse 3.8[20]

...but those
Who have discrimination, with a still mind
And a pure heart, reach journey's end,
Never again to fall into the jaws of death.

Commentary

In yoga therapy, therapists address both physical and mental issues, but are particularly interested in the psychological functions. Yoga

---

19 *The Upanishads*, 81.
20 *The Upanishads*, 81.

Yoga Therapy Theory

therapy also examines the conditions of rajas and tamas, the mental doshas as taught in Ayurveda. Most importantly, by training the charioteer (buddhi*)*, problems in the reins (manas) disappear. When the state described in this verse becomes the norm—having attained the discrimination necessary to achieve a still mind and pure heart—the mind is no longer disrupted and we are free from the cycle of birth and death (disease).

Yoga therapy aims for the realization of health based on such psycho-somatic functional theory, and for the purpose of training the buddhi, the discriminating intellect, instruction is provided in the three realms of body (asana), breath (pranayama) and mind (dhyana/meditation).

3) Human Functions as Explained in the Pancha Kosha and Human Chariot Theories

In the previous sections, I explained how five thousand years of wisdom from ancient India has culminated in giving us theories of human structure. Now I would like to explain how these models function. I will explain based primarily upon the pancha kosha theory with references to the human chariot theory (you may wish to refer back to Figures 1 and 2 in the previous section).

Annamaya Kosha

"Anna" means "food," and as its name suggests, the annamaya kosha is made from food. In the human chariot theory, the annamaya kosha is equivalent to the body of the chariot. If looked at from the perspective of conventional medicine, it is the physical body. Conventional medicine addresses illnesses that arise in this physical body, but according to the pancha kosha theory, causes of diseases that manifest in the physical body are disturbances that ripple up from deeper sheaths. Conventional medicine is very useful for emergency treatment of physical disorders, but the root causes are considered to be due to malfunctions at deeper levels, and yoga therapy has methods to correct these malfunctions. A yoga therapy approach to physical disorders in the annamaya kosha includes correcting or improving lifestyle, diet, and asana practice.

Pranamaya Kosha

This kosha is the sheath of vital energy, known in yoga as prana. Prana is not limited to this sheath, and has its origins in the Self, or *Atman*, the source of life itself; however, one of the grossest manifestations of prana in human functions is in the breath, which is closely related to the autonomic nervous system. From a medical perspective, disturbed breathing can be understood as autonomic nervous system disorders. Disorders of the autonomic nervous system disrupt endocrine and immune system functions, and these bring about the manifestation of diseases in the physical body. This mechanism was understood in ancient India, and this is now being addressed in the mind-body field of psychosomatic medicine. Both the annamaya kosha and pranamaya kosha are considered to be the body of the chariot in the chariot theory. To correct imbalances in the pranamaya kosha, breathing exercises called pranayama are used. There are more than one hundred pranayama techniques, but yoga therapy uses only ten techniques that do not easily lead to adverse events.

Manomaya Kosha

This kosha is comprised of the manas (mind), one of the four psychological organs, and the ten indriyas, often referred to as "sense organs." They are not physical organs, but are faculties of the mind-body. The ten indriyas include the five organs of perception (called jnana indriyas— seeing, hearing, touching, tasting, smelling) and the five organs of action (called karma indriyas—grasping, locomotion, reproduction, excretion, and speaking). In the human chariot theory, these ten indriyas are the ten horses, and the manas is the reins.

When these ten horses are out of control and do not function properly, the *Katha Upanishad* tells us that this leads to many lifestyle diseases and social problems. To ensure that the horses behave well, the *Yoga Sutras* introduce pratyahara, traditional practices to strengthen the manas's ability to control the senses. Yoga therapy has adapted simple pratyahara techniques to enable anyone to practice them.

Vijnanamaya Kosha

This kosha is comprised of the buddhi, another one of the four psychological organs, and is also known as intellect. This would be the charioteer. Whether the abovementioned reins (manas) control the ten horses skillfully or not is largely determined by the functions of the buddhi. Many of the psychosomatic, lifestyle, and stress-related disorders that conventional medicine is now struggling with, as well as psychological disorders like depression and eating disorders, are thought to have their origins in poor functioning of the vijnanamaya kosha. Traditional yoga puts the three practices of dharana (concentration), dhyana (meditation), and samadhi together into one category called samyama to correct malfunctions of the vijnanamaya kosha. Vedic meditation that utilizes the four steps of listening (shravana), contemplation (manana), deep meditation in daily life (nididhyasana), and realization/knowledge (jnana) is also important. These techniques are explained in more detail in the chapters on the vijnanamaya and anandamaya kosha in part III of this book.

Anandamaya Kosha

This kosha is comprised of the ahamkara, which creates the sense of self, and the chitta. These are the remaining two of the four psychological organs. The ahamkara is a psychological function that attaches a sense of self to various movements of the mind, such as when we say "I am..." or "mine." The chitta is a storehouse of memories. In traditional yoga, one of the goals is to make all of these memories healthy. In the first chapter of Patanjali's *Yoga Sutras*, yoga is defined as, "stilling the movement of the chitta."

The most troublesome memories in the chitta are known as trauma. Not only is their impact powerful, but we accumulate many of these and other unhealthy memories in the chitta from a very young age. Most of these memories are usually forgotten, but they still influence the way we see the world. I call them "forgotten memories." Though normally forgotten, they can be recalled with a little attention in meditation. Once aware of them, we can see the memories in a new light and understand them in a healthy way. This is a meditation technique, and it is among the final techniques used in yoga therapy instruction for healing people with psychosomatic and psychological disorders. For concrete examples, we introduce some case studies in this book, but for actual practice methods, it is necessary to receive instruction from a certified yoga therapist.

The preceding sections covered the pancha kosha and human chariot theories, explaining the structure of our mind-body complex. Next, I will introduce the theories of human structure and function as explained in Ayurveda, India's traditional medicine.

4) Ayurveda's Human Structure and Function Theories as Seen in the *Charaka Samhita*

Ayurveda's explanations of human structure and function are nearly identical to those of traditional yoga. Ayurveda also explains the methods for treating various diseases with different techniques based on its structural and function theories. As I explained earlier in this book, conventional medicine focuses primarily on the physical body, and uses anatomy as a structural theory, and physiology as a theory of the body's functions. These theories define what is normal or healthy. Diagnosis basically involves identifying differences in the client's condition in comparison to these standards, and treatment involves returning the client's condition to that of the standard. Ways to treat and restore structure and function

Yoga Therapy Theory

are constantly being improved. I will comment on some of the verses in the *Charaka Samhita* to give a simple explanation of how Ayurveda defines healthy structure and function and some of the methods of treatment.

Charaka Samhita Sharira Sthana, **Chapter I Verses 3–15**[21]

Agnivesa requested Punarvasu to explain the following:

1. *What are the divisions of the 'Empirical Soul' according to the division of* dhatus *(elements)?*
2. *Why is the 'Empirical Soul' considered to be the cause of the body?*
3. *What is the origin of 'Empirical Soul'?*
4. *Is 'Empirical Soul' a sentient or insentient object?*
5. *Is he eternal or ephemeral?*
6. *What is the primordial source of creation and what are its modifications?*
7. *What is the proof of the existence of the 'Empirical Soul'?*
8. *Those proficient in spiritual science describe the 'Empirical Soul' as devoid of action, independent, absolutely free, all pervasive, knower of the body and a witness. When is the 'Empirical Soul' devoid of action; how does action emanate from him?*
9. *If He is independent, how does he take birth among the undesirable species?*
10. *If He is absolutely free, how is He overpowered with miserable ideas?*
11. *Being omnipotent, is He not aware of all miseries?*
12. *If He is ubiquitous, how does He not visualize things interrupted by hills and walls?*
13. *Which comes first—the body or the knower of the body (Soul)?*
14. *In the absence of the knowable object in the form of the body, emergence of the 'Empirical Soul' as the body, does not appear to be appropriate. But then if the body comes first, the knower of the body i.e. the 'Empirical Soul' would lose its eternity.*

---

21 *Caraka Samhita* vol. II, 312.

15. *What is it of which the 'Empirical Soul' is considered to be a witness?*
16. *There is none else who could create things (one and the same 'Empirical Soul' cannot be a creator as well as a witness at the same time).*

    If the 'Empirical Soul' is derived from any modification, how does He subject himself to specific situations arising out of miseries (diseases)?
17–19. *Out of the three types of miseries of a patient, which one is treated by the physician—the past one, the present one or the future one? The future one is in fact not in existence; the past one has already ceased to exist and even the present one is, in a sense, momentary and so in the absence of continuity, it is not amenable to any treatment. So the above doubt about treatment is justifiable.*
20. *What are the causative factors of miseries (diseases)?*
21. *What are sites of their manifestation?*
22. *Where do all these miseries submerge after their cure?*
23. *What are the signs which help in the recognition of the 'Empirical Soul' which is omnipresent, all-renouncing, devoid of all contacts, only one and tranquil?*

Commentary

Is the Self a presence that has no movement but just watches everything? What is the source of this Self? What is its relationship with the *prakrti*, which is said to be the root of everything in the changing, material world? When a patient is ill, does the doctor work to heal the suffering of the past, present, or future? If the Self is the source of human existence, what aspect of the human is it the doctor's job to treat? These are the questions being raised in the above verses from the *Charaka Samhita*.

The tradition of Ayurveda is explained in what reads like a myth, in which a wise man named Bharadwaja went to heaven and learned Ayurveda from the god, Indra. Bharadwaja taught it to his disciple, Agnivesa, who then taught his disciple, Charaka. Regardless of the accuracy of this story, in Ayurveda, the realization of real health is unification with *Atman*, the source of human life. In Sanskrit, the word for health is *swasth*, or "self-existence." This word *swasth* apparently moved West to the Middle East, where it became *hasta*, and then again further west to become "health" in English.[22]

Because we do not identify ourselves with the Self (*Atman*), but tend to identify with things that are always changing—such as our bodies, states of mind, social status, and assets—we suffer from this misunderstanding of who we are. Charaka's teachings explain that doctors of Ayurveda heal patients of their mistaken identification. Ayurveda is not just treatment using medicated oils, massage, and herbal medicine, but it is a medical science to realize the immortal Self and attain spiritual liberation.

The concept of "Self" is too abstract to be of practical use in material conventional medicine, but we can understand Self to mean life itself. Life is an important concept in both medicine and in psychology, as indeed, there is no medical or psychological science that tries to heal corpses. *Ayur* means "life" and *veda* means "science," making it clear that Ayurveda is dealing with more than just the body. It examines the very question of life itself.

Sometimes patients receiving medical treatment complain that their doctors look only at the numbers from test results and do not look at the patients themselves as individual people. This means that there are doctors who do not look beyond the physical body to see the patient as an entire entity of life itself. Ayurveda is a medical science that looks at each patient as a whole.

---

22 D. B. Bisht, "Spiritual Dimensions of Health," in *Yoga Research and Applications: Proceedings of the 5ᵗʰ International Conference on Frontiers in Yoga Research and Applications*, ed. H. R. Nagendra, Shirley Telles (Bangalore, India: Vivekananda Kendra Yoga Research Foundation), (2000), 122.

Charaka Samhita Sharira Sthana Chapter I Verse 17[23]

According to another classification, Purusha *comprises twenty-four* dhatus, *i.e. mind, ten* indriyas *(sensory and motor organs), five objects of sense organs and* Prakrti *(consisting of eight* dhatus, *viz., five* mahabhutas *(in their subtle form),* ahamkara *(ego),* mahan *(intellect) and* avyakta *(primordial element).*

Commentary

In Ayurveda, the theory of human structure is based on twenty-four entities made from five elements, all of which envelop the Self. This theory may be very different from anatomy in conventional medicine, so Ayurveda should be valued for its theory and long history of treating many diseases, just as Chinese medicine is. In fact, it is said that Chinese medicine—with yin, yang, and five elements—evolved from Ayurveda as it moved east from India.

Charaka Samhita Sharira Sthana Chapter I Verses 18–19[24]

Sometimes, one understands a thing and sometimes one does not. This proves the existence of the mind as a separate sense organ. That is why, when there is no contact of the mind with the sense organs and their objects, no understanding of things can occur. It is only when the required mental contact is there, that one can understand things. Atomicity and oneness are considered to be the two characteristic features of the mind.

Commentary

In Ayurveda, the manas is the mind, the psychological organ that collects information from the outside world. It is equivalent to the

---

23 *Caraka Samhita,* vol. II, 314.
24 *Caraka Samhita,* vol. II, 315.

reins in the human chariot theory. In both Ayurveda and traditional yoga, the information that the indriyas (ten horses) collect is sent through the manas (mind/reins) to the buddhi (intellect). This information creates a stimulus that disrupts the cognitive and discriminative ability of the intellect (buddhi), and thus disrupts the functions of the entire human system. This is why it is important to correct the cognitive functions of the buddhi that handles this outside information. In Ayurveda and traditional yoga, the theories regarding functions of human structures are primarily concerned with assessment and correction of the discriminating intellect, that is, the functions of the buddhi.

Charaka Samhita Sharira Sthana Chapter I Verses 22–23[25]

Objects are perceived with the help of sense organs together with mind. This perception is purely mental in the beginning; the practical advantages or disadvantages are ascertained thereafter. The intellect which determines the specific properties of the object impels a (sane) individual to speak or act intelligently.

Commentary

Traditional yoga and Ayurveda are slightly different in how they differentiate between the functions of the mind and the intellect. In traditional yoga, the mind only receives information, and the intellect is what recognizes it, makes predictions and decisions, and gives orders for action. But however the division of labor is described, it is clear that Ayurveda also places importance on the psychological organs, and that it is these malfunctions which are the cause of disease. Even in conventional medicine, most people can understand how this would work in relation to stress-related psychosomatic and psychological disorders.

---

25 *Caraka Samhita*, vol. II, 317.

Kazuo Keishin Kimura

Charaka Samhita Sharira Sthana **Chapter I Verses 37–38**[26]

It is the combination of 24 elements known as Purusha, *action, fruit of action, knowledge, ignorance, happiness, misery, life, death and ownership are established. One who duly knows this, knows the life, death, continuity of the body, treatment (physical and spiritual) and all other knowable objects.*

Commentary

There is a very large difference in both daily life and life as a whole between those who view their state of mind objectively and those who get lost in their mental functions. Of the three types of treatment that Charaka discusses, two deal directly with promoting mental health, namely psychological and spiritual treatment. Yoga therapy also uses traditional Ayurvedic methods to promote mental health. One of these methods is to educate and guide the client to become free from the duality of pleasure and pain, life, and death.

Charaka Samhita Sharira Sthana **Chapter I Verse 53**[27]

As the Supreme Soul is beginningless, no birth as such can be ascribed to Him. Of course, the Empirical Soul (Purusha) *who represents the combination of 24 elements is born out of action prompted by likes and dislikes originated from ignorance.*

Commentary

This verse explains that the ultimate aim is to be free from our personal self, which we identify as the physical body and the four inner psychological organs. In traditional yoga, this is called

---

26 *Caraka Samhita*, vol. II, 321.
27 *Caraka Samhita*, vol. II, 325.

"ignorance" of our true nature, or our supreme Self. The ultimate medicine is to liberate the individualized self from this ignorance. In this verse, it is clear that Ayurveda is doing more than addressing physical ailments, and that traditional yoga plays a vital role in helping people attain the wisdom necessary not only for physical health, but for ultimate health.

Charaka Samhita Sharira Sthana **Chapter I Verses 75–76**[28]

Mind is active but devoid of consciousness. Thus the all-pervasive Soul while in combination with the mind appears to have actions. As the Soul has consciousness, it is said to be the agent of action. The mind being devoid of consciousness is said to be devoid of action even though it is possessed of action.

Commentary

In this verse, Charaka explains *Atman*, or the Self (translated earlier as "Soul"). The aim of traditional yoga is also realization of the Self, so it is not an exaggeration to say that what Ayurveda sees as the ultimate state of health is attainable with the practice of traditional yoga techniques. As Charaka says, the psychological organs (such as the manas and buddhi), are not conscious in and of themselves. They require consciousness to manifest, and we use these in yoga practices to deepen our experience of the Self. The Self, which is the source of all life, simply provides life energy, just as the rays of the sun shine and warm the earth, enabling the phenomenon of many life forms to go about their daily life activities. Just as the sun, the source of light and heat, does nothing itself to interfere in the various activities of the life forms on earth, the Self also provides life energy but does not interfere in the various physiological and psychological functions. Charaka was a physician,

---

28 *Caraka Samhita*, vol. II, 331.

but reading such verses, I am sure he also had abundant knowledge of traditional yoga.

Charaka Samhita Sharira Sthana Chapter I Verse 77[29]

All living beings join themselves on their own with life (elan vitae) in different species in accordance with the results of action performed. None else is responsible for the transmigration of living beings from one species to another.

Commentary

In both traditional yoga and Ayurveda, the efficient cause of the universe is the life-principle, which has several names. Sometimes it is called, *Atman, Paramatman,* or *Purusha.* In traditional yoga, the purpose of life is to reach this pure, source of all life. In Ayurveda as well, the role of the doctor is to guide the patient to this pure Life Principle. This is why Charaka says that not only is rational treatment (using medicines and other techniques for the body) necessary, but that psychological and spiritual treatments are also essential.

Charaka Samhita Sharira Sthana Chapter I Verse 78[30]

The Soul is absolutely free to act as he pleases. He is however obliged to enjoy the fruits of his own action. He is also free to control his mind and to get rid of the results of good or bad acts of his own.

Commentary

It is said that *Atman* itself does not act. If it took action, it would be necessary for *Atman* to change, and it would no longer be possible to say that *Atman* is an eternal and never-changing presence. But because it is the cause of all action, it sees the

---

29 *Caraka Samhita*, vol. II. 331.
30 *Caraka Samhita*, vol. II, 331.

results of all changes in creation. Yoga is turning attention to the Self, and unification with the Self is called samadhi. This state of samadhi is a state completely free from the changing material world. Yoga therapy also seeks to take clients to this state. Yoga therapy is not limited to the physical realm of posture or strength training.

Above, I have briefly introduced the theories of human structure and function according to yoga and Ayurveda, and shown how they are fundamentally the same. In the following section, I will introduce how Charaka explains the role of the physician, because yoga therapists should also take this to heart when working with clients.

5) The Role of Physicians as Explained in the *Charaka Samhita*

Based on the above theories of human structure and function, Charaka explains some things for physicians to keep in mind. In the verses that follow, "physician" can also be read as "yoga therapist." What he explains for physicians is relevant to yoga therapists as well.

Charaka Samhita Vimanasthana Chapter VIII Verse 3[31]

A wise man, desirous of adopting medical profession should, first of all, carefully select a suitable text on medicine, depending upon his competence to undertake light or serious type of work, his willingness for short term or long term results, his habitat and age. There are several such texts available for physicians. Only the texts having the following characteristic features are to be followed:

1. *Which are followed by great, illustrious and wise physicians (for those texts which are great and popular and are followed by wise persons.)*
2. *Which are pregnant with ideas and respected by reputed experts;*

---

31 *Caraka Samhita*, vol. II, 215.

3. Which are conducive to the intellectual growth of disciples of all the three categories (viz., highly intelligent, moderately intelligent and less intelligent);
4. Which are free from defects of repetition, transmitted by seers and have well-knit aphorisms together with commentaries thereon in proper order;
5. Which have elegant ideas to convey;
6. Which are free from vulgar and difficult expressions and have clear and unambiguous expressions;
7. Which convey ideas in an orderly manner;
8. Which primarily deal with the determination of real objects;
9. Which are free from contradictions;
10. Where there is no confusion relating to contexts;
11. Which convey ideas quickly; and
12. Which are equipped with definitions (of etiology, symptomatology and therapeutics) and illustrations. A text of this type may be compared to the sun which removes darkness and illuminates all.

Commentary

What Charaka says in this verse is still relevant and applicable to medical doctors today. In yoga therapy as well, it is clear from this verse that we need an accurate theory for instruction in addition to case study reports that help us to understand the mechanism for restoration of health. That is to say, the yoga therapist should, on the basis of the pancha kosha and human chariot theories, understand the ideal human state, and then assess the functions of the client's vijnanamaya and anandamaya koshas for any problems. Based on that assessment, yoga therapists can help the client restore the vijnanamaya and anandamaya koshas to a healthy state. We still need more case studies to back up this theory for instruction, but the Japan Yoga Therapy Society holds annual research conferences in which such valuable information is being collected and many case studies are being presented.

Charaka Samhita Vimanasthana **Chapter VIII Verse 4**[32]

Therefore one should assess the qualities of the preceptor. An ideal preceptor is he who is well grounded in scriptures; equipped with practical knowledge, wise, skillful, whose prescriptions are infallible, who is pious, who has all the necessary equipment for treatment, who is not deficient in respect of any of the sense organs, who is acquainted with human nature, and the rationale of treatment, whose knowledge is not overshadowed by the knowledge of other scriptures, who is free from vanity, envy and anger, who is hard working, who is affectionately disposed towards his disciples and is capable of expressing his views with clarity. A preceptor possessed of such qualities infuses medical knowledge to a good disciple as the seasonal cloud helps bring about good crop in a fertile land.

Commentary

In Ayurveda, a skillful physician is one who possesses accurate knowledge of the ideal human structure and function and who can diagnose the defects in a person's body and mind based on this knowledge. Such physicians also possess the skills to return patients to the ideal structure and function, and are able to teach their disciples.

In the case of yoga therapy, yoga therapists must study the traditional scriptures in order to understand the ideal conditions of the manomaya, vijnanamaya, and anandamaya koshas. This understanding is crucial in Ayurvedic psychological and spiritual treatments. Yoga therapists also need to understand the functions of the psychological doshas of rajas, tamas, and sattva. Based on this, the therapist assesses how the psychological functions of rajas and tamas are functioning in the client, and at

---

32 *Caraka Samhita*, vol. II, 217.

the same time, must be adept in using yoga therapy techniques to return the mental doshas to a healthy state. Charaka is also saying that to become skilled in applying the techniques of yoga therapy requires being instructed by a skillful therapist with these superior skills.

Charaka Samhita Sharira Sthana Chapter I Verse 86–94[33]

> *The principle on which the treatment of diseases pertaining to the past, present and future is based, is as follows;*
>
> *Recurrence of headache, fever, cough and vomiting establishes the fact that diseases of the past do relapse. That is to say, the tie of occurrence of the various diseases in the past repeats itself. The therapeutic devices meant for alleviating such recurring diseases verily take the past history (of such diseases) into consideration.*
>
> *In order that flood waters may not damage crops as they did in the past, a dam is constructed as a preventive measure. So are some therapeutic devices prescribed to prevent certain diseases which are likely to attack living beings in future. This treatment relates to prevention of future diseases.*
>
> *The successive continuity of ailments is checked by treatments conducive to the continuity of happiness.*
>
> *The state of equilibrium of* dhatus *is not disturbed nor is the imbalanced state brought to normalcy without some causative factors. It is the causative factors which determine the equilibrium or imbalance of the dhatus.*
>
> *So a physician treats the diseases pertaining to the past, present and future.*

Commentary

In the case of treating modern illnesses, conventional medicine is struggling to deal with psychosomatic and lifestyle diseases, the

---

33 *Caraka Samhita*, vol. II, 335.

causes of which are often hidden in the client's lifestyle or belief systems regarding how to live. Most people are aware that continued intake of unhealthy food or continuing unhealthy habits will eventually lead to manifestation of disease in the body. Most people need to reconsider and correct beliefs and habits that lead to physical illness. In modern society, one group of people who are in a position to do something about this are yoga therapists. I hope that what is introduced in this book will also be useful for yoga therapists to practice and incorporate into their own lives.

Following are the last words of Charaka that I would like to introduce in this chapter.

Charaka Samhita Indriyasthana Chapter I Verse 5[34]

Natural disposition is of six categories depending upon the distinctive feature of;
    1. Caste…2. Family…3. Locality…4. Time…5. Age of the patient… 6. The individual.

Commentary

Yoga therapists are well suited to address psychological health as understood in Ayurveda, and from this perspective, they must be aware of family medical history, upbringing, and lifestyle. They also need to know the client's medical history, current condition, and assess the risks for future problems. For this purpose, therapists need to have the knowledge and ability to assess clients' mental *doshas* and how they may be disrupting psychological functions. Therapists must also know what kinds of environments clients are living in, and the ideal psychological models for those environments. With this knowledge, assessments become more refined.

---

34 *Caraka Samhita*, vol. II, 520.

As described earlier, in both conventional medicine as well as in yoga therapy, the quality of medical diagnosis or assessment is crucial. The level of skill in helping clients restore their health will depend greatly on the depth of wisdom that the doctors or yoga therapists possess. With regard to yoga therapy instruction, yoga therapists advise clients on yoga therapy techniques that the clients must practice themselves. They simply provide recommendations for practices, and this is why we consider the therapist as a counselor. In the case of yoga therapy, we do not call it "treatment" but call it yoga therapy instruction. Patients must be active in their own healing to heal the diseases that they create themselves. The yoga therapist's role is only to assist.

The yoga therapist's role may only be to assist clients in self-healing, but they have much to offer the world. Just as people have family doctors, I believe it would be ideal for people to have a "family yoga therapist" who is familiar with their history over an extended period of time.

PART II

Yoga Therapy in Practice:
Yoga Therapy Assessment (YTA)

CHAPTER 1

Yoga Therapy Principles

for Assessment and Instruction

THOSE WHO ARE READING THIS book for help in addressing mind-body imbalance, feel free to skip to part II. It is important reading, however, for people teaching yoga. It will become clear why it is essential that instructors conduct an assessment of clients and students prior to yoga instruction. It is important to remember that in spite of the fact that yoga therapy classes are not medical clinics, many people with various kinds of disorders are looking to yoga for help. Keeping this in mind, it is best to conduct an intake for all new students or clients along the lines of the procedures I explain in this chapter.

1) THE SIX STAGES IN YOGA THERAPY

STAGE I: YOGA THERAPY ASSESSMENT (YTA)

The first step in yoga therapy is the assessment. Yoga therapists must first conduct an intake interview, and then obtain the client's informed consent for both the content and duration of instruction. These procedures are very important.

Yoga therapy requires that clients are assessed in accordance with all the sheaths of human existence—that is, the five koshas. Physical assessment should be conducted, but assessment of the deeper layers of a person's existence holds the key to fundamental healing. Yoga teaches that disease has its root causes in malfunction of the discriminating intellect, and that this disruption eventually manifests as disease in the physical body.

In cases where the client has already been diagnosed with a disorder by a medical or Ayurvedic doctor, it is necessary for the yoga therapist to be informed of this, and then to assess the function of the buddhi. Yoga therapy can be considered a modality of psychotherapy using techniques that address both body and mind. I will explain the assessment of the manomaya and vijnanamaya koshas in chapters III and IV of part III of this book. To facilitate assessment of these koshas, the Japan Yoga Therapy Society has developed several semi-structured interview manuals (SSIM). They provide a framework of questions with a scoring system that therapists can use in their initial intake interviews with clients to assess their mental conditions and provide a reference to measure changes in the clients' condition as therapy progresses. Following are the names of some of the interview manuals and questionnaires that we have developed.

- Semi-Structured Interview Manual: Yoga Sutra-Based State of Mind Assessment (SSIM-YSSMA) (for yoga therapists use)
- Semi-Structured Interview Manual: Yoga Sutra-Based Assessment of Misrecognition (SSIM-YSAM) (for yoga therapists' use)
- Semi-Structured Interview Manual: *Bhagavad Gita*-based Assessment of Karma (SSIM-BGAK) (for yoga therapists' use)
- Ayurvedic Psychological Dosha Assessment (APDA) (for clients' use)

To assess the anandamaya kosha:

- Semi-Structured Interview Manual: Assessment of Spirituality (SSIM-AS) (for yoga therapists' use)

Yoga Therapy Theory

An example of an assessment tool from India:

- sVYASA General Health Questionnaire, made by the Swami Vivekananda Yoga Anusandhana Samasthana in Bengaluru, India.

Before using these interview manuals and questionnaires, it is important that yoga therapists are clear on precisely what they want to assess, as this will determine which assessment tool to use. Different assessment tools examine different aspects of the psychological condition, so they must be selected carefully. This is particularly true when using the more specialized psychological tests used in clinical psychology, such as the following:

- POMS (Profile of Mood States)
- STAI (State-Trait Anxiety Inventory)
- Yatabe–Guilford Personality Test (YGPI)

These psychological tests are easy to use for yoga therapists even if they have not been professionally educated in psychology. When using these questionnaires, however, the therapist must first receive the client's informed consent, as the results of the tests need to be shared with the client in a way that dispels unnecessary doubt but does not create unnecessary worry. Please be aware that reading this book is not sufficient training to know how to use these tests.

In order to understand the condition of a client's stress, the stress-coping inventory and other inventories may be considered for use. In addition, through counseling, it is also possible to assess the meaning clients have given to various life events and what attachments they have. In particular, it is important to hear from clients concretely about emotional life events and what they think about those events. In this way, it is possible to identify characteristics and patterns in their way of thinking.

STAGE 2: SELECTING YOGA THERAPY TECHNIQUES

After assessing where problems are arising in the human system (the five koshas), yoga therapists consider what needs to be done to address the problems. In other words, they create a plan for yoga therapy instruction and choose the techniques to use. In medicine, this might be called "treatment." In yoga therapy, one of the underlying principles is that clients have created their own disorders, be it digestive ulcers, high blood pressure, or cancer, and that they can address those problems themselves, in consultation with a yoga therapist. So we do not use the term "treatment" at JYTS. Treatment implies that the client is a recipient of a medicine or procedure, but in yoga therapy, the client is the most active practitioner. We believe that yoga therapy teaches clients to take their health into their own hands, and their yoga therapy practice facilitates empowerment and enhances their natural healing capacities by addressing the necessary defective areas of the five koshas.

I introduce some yoga therapy techniques in various sections of this book, so I would like to list here which techniques are primarily used for each kosha.

* *Annamaya kosha*: asana and other physical practices
* *Pranamaya kosha*: simple breathing exercises (*pranayama*)
* *Manomaya kosha*: techniques to control the senses (*pratyahara*)
* *Vijnanamaya kosha*: meditation instruction, such as Vedic meditation
* *Anandamaya kosha*: meditation instruction, such as Vedic meditation.

The yoga therapist must understand the mechanism of how health is recovered to create effective yoga therapy programs. Every year, new research papers are being published about how yoga therapy works in various areas, such as immunology and brain function, so yoga therapists must be diligent in keeping up with the most recent research. The results of medical and yoga therapy research should also be considered and incorporated into yoga therapy. Later, I will explain more about the mechanism of how yoga therapy can help restore health in simple terms so that people who are not yet yoga therapists can also understand easily. It is common sense that no matter what the area of expertise, continued learning is important. Yoga and yoga therapy are no different.

We are also in the process of making yoga therapy instruction guidelines for specific ailments, because we see this as an urgent need in the field of yoga therapy.

STAGE 3: YOGA THERAPY INSTRUCTION (INDIVIDUAL, GROUP AND SYMPTOM-BASED)

After selecting the yoga techniques to use in yoga therapy, practice is of course essential. There are various ways in which this can be done.

In India, some hospitals have yoga therapy departments, and doctors refer patients to them just as they would refer them to surgery or any other department. In situations like this, it is impossible to provide instruction for everyone at one time in a group lesson, because there is a vast array of patients diagnosed with different illnesses. For example, if a pregnant woman goes to the yoga therapy department at the hospital at the same time as someone with rheumatoid arthritis, it is clear that they have very different needs and should not receive the same yoga therapy practice. This is why yoga therapy is, in principle, designed for each individual. But in yoga classes around the world, we are seeing increasing numbers of people with various disorders joining classes where everyone is taught the same thing regardless. In such circumstances, adverse events are bound to arise. I have not, however, found academic papers written about adverse events in yoga, other than the study I mentioned at the beginning of this book conducted in 2013 by researchers at Kyushu University's Graduate School of Medical Science. To prevent adverse events, it is best to provide personalized instruction to clients who are addressing specific problems.

When I first went to the Kaivalyadhama Yoga Institute in Lonavla, Maharashtra, in the 1970s, I was able to observe how yoga therapy was instructed there. All patients doing yoga therapy had their own chart with an individualized program. Though many people were practicing yoga in the same room at the same time, each patient did their own practice under the supervision of a yoga therapist. Such individualized instruction was also being carried out in the yoga therapy department of Banaras Hindu University Institute of Medical Science, as well as at the Mumbai University Faculty of Medicine, and other yoga therapy departments all over India.

In addition to personalized practice, there is also symptom-based instruction. This type of instruction is done at the Swami Vivekananda Yoga Research Foundation, where they have a yoga therapy facility called Prashanti Kutiram ("Place of Peace"). They provide yoga therapy instruction there throughout the year. There are a few medical doctors there, as well as many yoga therapists, and tens of thousands of patients have benefited from their services. Lessons are divided into categories such as yoga for people with cardiovascular disorders, diabetes, and obesity. Patients are divided based on their medical diagnosis, and the yoga therapists who work there instruct from early in the morning until night. During that time, there are also prayer times for psychoeducation, and time to study about diseases themselves. The yoga therapy facility is located in a large area in the suburbs of Bengaluru where the inpatient facility and yoga university is located. The patients come from both India and abroad. There are also ongoing yoga instructor and yoga therapist training courses. In recent years, the training courses have become very international, attracting students from all around the world, including mainland China.

The most common type of yoga instruction in the world today is grouping both healthy and unhealthy people together in the same yoga lesson and having them all practice the same techniques. In such cases, one instructor may teach dozens of students. Recently in India, we are seeing thousands of people taught together, including people with

Yoga Therapy Theory

various illnesses, and such manner of instruction is spreading. It is very different from the individualized or symptom-based instruction I explained earlier.

Such large-group instruction creates a situation where many people with varying degrees of mental and physical health and severity of symptoms are given exactly the same practice. Invariably, that practice is going to be unsuitable for some, and adverse events during such classes are unsurprisingly common. If you find yourself as an instructor in this kind of situation, keep students with the most serious symptoms and those who need the most attention as close to you as possible. When necessary, instruct them to do things differently from the rest of the class. For example, a woman in her eighth month of pregnancy, an elderly person, or someone of limited mobility with rheumatoid arthritis may need extra attention.

As mentioned earlier, yoga therapists must be ready and able to adjust instruction based on how the yoga therapy assessment defines the needs of the client. As public medical and social welfare institutions become more interested in yoga therapy, therapists must keep in mind the importance of personalized instruction as the most desirable type of instruction in order to prevent adverse events.

STAGE 4: MONITORING CHANGES IN THE CLIENT'S CONDITION (CCC) USING YOGA-BASED TOOLS

Once yoga therapy instruction commences based on a yoga therapy assessment, it is necessary to observe and record what kinds of changes the client is feeling and whether the content of instruction is in fact restoring and promoting health. This is important because the observations and records are the documents referred to when determining if the content of instruction is succeeding and if it requires change. The following can be used to document and compare the changes in the client's condition (CCC) before and after yoga therapy instruction.

- Subjective data (client's narrative)
- Changes in results of the SSIM-YSAM, SSIM-BGAK, or other YTA tools

STAGE 5: EXAMINING CHANGES IN THE CLIENT'S CONDITION (CCC) USING DATA FROM CONVENTIONAL MEDICINE AND CLINICAL PSYCHOLOGY

It is necessary to examine the effects of yoga therapy programs in light of assessments from clinical psychology as well as changing medical data. Medical institutions now provide clients with printed information that contains the pharmacological names of the medicine they have been prescribed, as well as copies of various test results. Yoga therapists who are not medical professionals should be careful not to criticize or object to doctors' decisions and treatment. If clients report feeling changes in their conditions, or changes are indicated by medical data, it is important for yoga therapists to consider this information and decide if the yoga therapy programs are appropriate or not.

If a client's condition worsens, it is necessary to reexamine the content of the yoga therapy program. If the client is responding well to both the yoga therapy program and medical treatment, it is also important to decide whether to continue the same yoga therapy techniques or to change the content of the program to match the changes in the client's condition to improve health further. This is why it is important to examine the results of various tests over time. In this way, yoga therapists can respect and refer to the expertise of other health professionals while providing yoga therapy instruction.

STAGE 6: TRANSITIONING FROM YOGA THERAPY TO TRADITIONAL YOGA

Recovery of physical health is not the end of yoga therapy. Charaka explained that complete emancipation is the ultimate well-being. After clients regain physical well-being, yoga therapists should facilitate improved mental capacity and mental health, guiding the client to a higher dimension so that psychosomatic illnesses do not recur. To do this, clients should progress from yoga therapy to traditional yoga practice. Through traditional Raja Yoga instruction, a yoga therapist can guide a client to develop further as a human being. This is why it is essential for yoga therapists to study not only yoga therapy but also study traditional yoga and themselves strive toward the ultimate state of well-being and share this wisdom while instructing their clients.

To summarize, yoga therapy begins with the assessment (YTA), then based on this assessment, techniques are chosen for yoga therapy instruction (YTI), which is done while monitoring the changes in the client's condition (CCC) as the client continues to practice. Finally, once a degree of health is reached, the client should transition into traditional yoga practice.

In the next section, I explain more about traditional yoga practice that therapists should incorporate into their own daily practices to improve their skills in assessment and instruction.

CHAPTER 2

Discerning the Unreal from the Real and

Yoga Therapy Assessment (YTA)

IN JAPAN, IT IS OFTEN said that the world is a reflection of our own minds. This means that our perception of the world and other people is based on how our minds interpret the world around us. It is, therefore, essential that yoga therapists cultivate inner wisdom to accurately assess clients' physical and mental conditions. As experts, yoga therapists must constantly purify and sharpen their intellect and be aware of their own criteria and standards for judgment.

In other words, yoga therapists should understand what comprises an ideal state of psychological health in terms of the vijnanamaya and anandamaya koshas. With this understanding, they can cultivate their ability to accurately assess the degree of predominance of mental doshas creating mental imbalance (rajas and tamas), in accordance with Ayurvedic teachings. In order to evaluate another's psychological condition, the person doing the evaluating must be as close as possible to the ideal sattvic condition. For this purpose, yoga therapists must consistently practice traditional yoga by, for example, studying ancient yoga scriptures or listening to the discourse of respected teachers. It is also absolutely essential that therapists have their own meditation practice, which we call *yoga sadhana*. Yoga therapists should, as Charaka says, strive to sharpen their own ability to distinguish between the real Self and what is misidentification (self-image). To do this, practicing traditional Raja Yoga is essential.

One example of when this skill is important is evident in JYTS's work in Thailand, providing yoga therapy instruction to people with drug addictions. Some of the participants in the program have voiced anger about their living environment. Essentially, they are mourning the difference between who they wanted to become and who they think they are. Both are misunderstandings of the truth of what they really are.

In Thailand, there is an expression, "mentality of retired people" to describe how someone who was the president of a large company, for example, gets angry when treated as a weak, elderly person with no particular social status. This is also an example of how even as a society, there is awareness of how people hold mistaken identities. Raja Yoga enables people to objectively see the falseness of the identities they have created for themselves and correct their understanding.

Now I will explain a little bit about yoga therapy assessment based on Patanjali's *Yoga Sutras* and the *Bhagavad Gita*. This kind of study enables yoga therapists to understand what comprises the ideal standard for physical and mental health based on ancient texts, and how to assess the abnormalities in clients' psychological functions. This is the same as a medical doctor identifying the defects of the physical body, such as high blood pressure or defective liver functions, based on what has been set as the standard health indicators in physiology. For this reason, study and understanding of the traditional yoga scriptures is essential not only for ascetics practicing Raja Yoga, but for yoga therapists.

1) YOGA THERAPY ASSESSMENT (YTA) AND PATANJALI'S *YOGA SUTRAS*

The *Yoga Sutras* of Patanjali are widely known as the fundamental text for yoga. The *Yoga Sutras* explain the eight limbs of yoga, the purpose of which is purification through to the chitta, the storehouse of memories. Psychological functions are divided into categories, and the *Yoga Sutras* provide teachings that enable us to assess and purify these functions, and provide a definition of perfect health. I will introduce some of these verses that follow.

As I mentioned previously, there is significant overlap between the *Yoga Sutras* and Charaka's teachings on Ayurveda. They overlap so much that some people speculate that Patanjali and Charaka were the same person. The *Yoga Sutras* are comprised of four chapters, and in this section, I will provide commentary on practical verses from chapters 1 and 2. They contain verses that also offer more concrete explanations for some of the concepts introduced in the *Charaka Samhita*. In a sense, these verses can be considered the "physiology" of yoga therapy. To truly understand, it is essential to study Raja Yoga under an experienced and knowledgeable teacher, so please simply read and do not practice what is written here without guidance.

Yoga Sutras Chapter 1 *Samadhi Pada* Verse 2

Yoga is the inhibition of the modifications of the mind (chitta).

Commentary

Chitta is the storehouse of memory, and in Verse 1.11, Patanjali explains memory as "not allowing an object which has been experienced to escape." If this is read together with what is written in verse 2, yoga can be considered a way to attain a state where psychological faculties, including memory, are no longer disrupted or disturbed.

Everyone has many memories going all the way back to the beginning of their lives, and among these, the memories that are most likely to cause illness are repressed trauma-related memories. Traditional yogic practices help to educate practitioners and purify mental functions so that even these trauma-related memories are no longer disruptive. A person who has not received such psychoeducation is likely to make erroneous judgments when handling the stresses of modern society, and is therefore particularly susceptible to developing psychosomatic and stress-related disorders. It is the role of yoga therapists to notice superficial symptoms, such as expressions of anger or panic, assess them, and work with clients to identify forgotten memories and to work toward healthier cognition of those memories that are at the root of the problems.

Yoga Sutras Chapter 1 *Samadhi Pada* Verse 3

Then the Seer is established in his own nature.

Commentary

Through yoga's various techniques, it is possible to attain a state of consciousness in which our psychological faculties remain undisturbed by any memories we have. In such a state, our mental and physical condition is a direct reflection of our essential nature of the Self, the innermost life principle. Today, we sometimes talk of athletes being "in the zone" or artists giving a divinely inspired performance. These are examples of such direct reflection of the Self, "established in its own nature." This was understood more than two thousand years ago by yogis and was recorded by Patanjali. We can also live in a way that is established in unity so that our daily mental and physical states reflect the truth of the Self.

Yoga Sutras Chapter 1 *Samadhi Pada* Verse 4

Otherwise, it conforms itself to the mental process

Commentary

Of the four inner psychological organs, chitta is the storehouse of memories. If many memories are accumulated as a result of disturbed psychological functions, then it can only be expected that mental functions emerging from such memories are also going to be disturbed. Modern psychology is also making clear how disturbed states of mind can lead to other disorders and illnesses in the body as well, but this verse from two thousand years ago had already made this body-mind connection. Mental functions that are ingrained though one's upbringing and living environment become habitual, and if a person is unable to observe themselves objectively, they mistakenly identify themselves as these mental functions. It is the job of the yoga therapist or yoga instructor to assess whether the client has such misunderstanding.

*Yoga Sutra*s Chapter 1 *Samadhi Pada* Verse 5

The modifications of the mind are five-fold and are painful or not-painful.

Commentary

Traditional yoga divides memory into five categories, as explained in verse 4 earlier. Each category can be subdivided into memories that cause suffering or do not cause suffering. Of India's religions, Japanese people are most familiar with Buddhism, in which there are 108 types of such afflictions. In traditional yoga, there are five. From the point of view of yoga therapy, to assess a client's painful mental processes, it is easier to use yoga's five categories. The teachings in yoga are very practical and are clear and simple enough for anyone to understand.

*Yoga Sutra*s Chapter 1 *Samadhi Pada* Verse 6

(They are) Right knowledge, wrong knowledge, fancy, sleep, and memory.

Commentary

Each of the five modifications of the *chitta* have two categories of those that are afflicted and cause pain, or those that do not. This gives us a total of ten modifications of the chitta. I will not explain them in detail in this book, but speaking from the perspectives of psychosomatic medicine and yoga therapy, this verse can be understood to be saying that the modifications of the chitta—right knowledge, wrong knowledge, imagination, sleep, and memory—are also the causes of disturbance of the buddhi, the psychological organ that comprises the faculties of intellect and sensitivity.

Yoga therapy is the process of assessing how the afflicted modifications are functioning within the client, and then instructing the client in techniques to restore the chitta to a healthy state. This is what we call YTA and YTI. There are many people with various illnesses going to yoga classes all over the world, so yoga instructors also need to educate themselves about these fundamental principles of yoga therapy.

Yoga Sutras Chapter 1 *Samadhi Pada* Verse 30

Disease, languor, doubt, carelessness, laziness, worldly-mindedness, delusion, non-achievement of a stage, instability, these (nine) cause the distraction of the mind and they are the obstacles.

Commentary

According to Patanjali's *Yoga Sutras*, there are nine causes for disturbance of the *chitta*, and they are obstacles to self-realization. Practitioners of traditional yoga do not practice for health reasons but are striving to stop the fluctuation of the chitta so that the pure consciousness of the true Self is able to manifest without distortion, directly through the body and mind. This ultimate liberation, or complete union, is called *moksha*. If moksha is used as the standard for ideal health, the condition of patients with stress-related and psychosomatic illnesses is far from ideal.

Patanjali explains that there are nine types of disturbed mental states that are obstacles to moksha. These nine states can be used in yoga therapy assessments, and JYTS has organized them into the *Semi-Structures Interview Manual: Yoga Sutra–Based State of Mind Assessment (SSIM-YSSMA)*, a manual that can be used by yoga therapists to interview and assess their clients. Once the causes for disturbance in the client's mind can be identified, it is then necessary to provide the best yoga therapy practices that will help to quieten the mind. Techniques are included in chapter 2 of the *Yoga Sutras*, and I will introduce a few of them next.

Yoga Sutras Chapter 2 *Sadhana Pada* Verse 5

> *Avidya is taking the non-eternal, impure, evil and non-Atman to be eternal, pure, good and Atman respectively.*

Commentary

While *Yoga Sutras* Verse 1.30 lists causes of mental disturbances such as apathy and doubt, there is a deeper cause, which is explained in this verse. Ignorance of the Self, or wrong cognition, is said to be the fundamental cause of all suffering. In yoga therapy, it is very important to assess the four kinds of wrong understanding explained in this verse. At JYTS, we developed a YTA tool for therapists to use called the *Semi-Structured Interview Manual for the Yoga Sutra-Based Assessment of Misrecognitions* (SSIM-YSAM), and therapists in Japan use this. In order to overcome the misunderstandings caused by ignorance, clients need to develop intellectual faculties and the sensitivity to be aware of their own cognition. In yoga therapy instruction, there are many methods to help develop this ability to see things more objectively. Further explanations of these methods are introduced briefly in various parts of this book.

Yoga Sutras Chapter 2 *Sadhana Pada* Verse 28

From the practice of the component exercises of Yoga, on the destruction of impurity, arises spiritual illumination that develops into awareness of Reality.

Commentary

Concrete traditional yoga practices come from the four great schools of yoga, namely, Raja Yoga, Jnana Yoga, Karma Yoga, and Bhakti Yoga. In this verse, however, with the phrase "component exercises of yoga," Patanjali is referring to the eight limbs of Raja Yoga (known as *ashtanga yoga*)—namely, yama, niyama, asana, pranayama, pratyahara, dharana, dhyana, and samadhi. Yoga therapy has adapted these eight limbs of Raja Yoga. I will introduce some samples of the techniques in following chapters.

From this verse, it is evident that Raja Yoga is a discipline to eliminate the ignorance that leads to misrecognition (of the non-eternal as eternal, etc.), so Raja Yoga can be considered an educational system that takes people to the ultimate goal of moksha, where there is complete independence from anything material. First, the mind is assessed for misrecognition. Then through practice of the eight limbs of Raja Yoga, the mind is purified all the way to the functions of the chitta, until moksha is achieved. This is also the aim of yoga therapy as psychoeducation. In the following chapters of this book, I will introduce yoga therapy assessment and practices for each kosha, beginning with the annamaya kosha (food sheath).

2) Yoga Therapy Assessment (YTA) and The *Bhagavad Gita*

Legend has it that the sage, Vyasa, compiled the four Vedas, and in order to make the teachings more accessible to laypeople, he told the epic story of the Mahabharata. He was also a yogi. In the Mahabharata, one part is known as the *Bhagavad Gita*, and it explains human action. A personality inventory based on the *Bhagavad Gita* was developed in India and the United States. There is also the Vedic personality inventory by David Wolf.

* *The Gita-Inventory of Personality*, by R. C. Das, Salt Lake City, *Journal of Indian Psychology* 9, Nos. 1 and 2 (1991).
* *The Vedic Personality Inventory*, by Dr. David Wolf

JYTS has also developed a semi-structured interview manual based on the *Bhagavad Gita* for use by yoga therapists.

* *Semi-Structured Interview Manual, Bhagavad Gita–Based Assessment of Karma* (SSIM-BGAK).

Our SSIMs are available for use only by yoga therapists who have undergone professional training and have been certified by JYTS.

REFERENCE 1: *BHAGAVAD GITA*

The *Bhagavad Gita* contains many standards that can be used to assess the human mind, because it is a story about the basic principles of action. Just before a great battle, General Arjuna hesitates to order his soldiers to attack when he sees old friends and relatives lined up on the other side. The divine Krishna instructs Arjuna in the principles of action, so the *Bhagavad Gita* is also known as a text on Karma Yoga (yoga of action). Of all human actions, the action of taking the life of another human being is the most confusing and difficult, even in cases of war in modern society. It is for this reason that the death penalty is still debated, and why people around the world are protesting war as a means to resolve conflict. This is true particularly after we experienced two world wars. It is natural that Arjuna, who is faced with battle and bloodshed, hesitates to order his troops to begin battle. But Krishna, who had taken on the appearance of Arjuna's chariot driver, sees Arjuna's confusion and explains the various states of the human mind. Krishna then tells Arjuna to issue the order to begin battle. In the eighteenth and final chapter of the *Bhagavad Gita*, Arjuna recovers his resolve to fight and orders his soldiers to advance.

This scripture is not about whether or not war is justifiable, but is about how people should fulfill their duties. Every day, we are faced with decisions on important actions. How do we perceive our responsibilities, and what decisions do we make that become the basis for action? The *Bhagavad Gita*, which was written several thousand years ago, is still considered to hold answers today. In India, wisdom that transcends space and time is called *sanatana dharma*, which means "eternal and unchanging order of the universe." The *Bhagavad Gita* is an example of this, having gone beyond change in time and place.

At JYTS, we used the *Bhagavad Gita* to develop yoga therapy assessment tools. I would like to introduce some passages that are useful for assessing clients, as they explain how the human mind works.

Bhagavad Gita Chapter 16 Verses 1–5 "The Divine and Demonic Natures"

Verse 1: *The Blessed Lord said: 1. Fearlessness, purity of heart, steadfastness in Yoga and knowledge, alms-giving,* *control of the senses, sacrifice, study of scriptures, austerity and straightforwardness,*

Verse 2: *Harmlessness, truth, absence of anger, renunciation, peacefulness, absence of crookedness, compassion toward beings, uncovetousness, gentleness, modesty, absence of fickleness,*

Verse 3: *Vigour, forgiveness, fortitude, purity, absence of hatred, absence of pride—these belong to one born in a divine state, O Arjuna!*

Commentary: As explained in the preceding verses and the ones that follow, there are people in this world born in "divine states" and "demonical states." Krishna explains this to Arjuna and teaches him what actions must be taken by someone with divine qualities. For us, living in modern, stressful societies, we are exposed to a lot of information every day and have to make decisions. Even if not to the degree of severity of Arjuna, who had to decide whether or not to wage war, we could consider ourselves in the same situation. Of course, it is most desirable to be in as noble a state of mind as possible in our daily lives, but most people cannot do this. The current reality is that there are a lot of people who are falling ill with various stress-related illnesses.

It is for this reason that the Bhagavad Gita, as a Karma Yoga scripture, is so useful for yoga therapy assessment. It is a text that has been used for thousands of years as a foundation to assess people's mental conditions, so it is undeniably worth lending an ear to the teachings. Yoga therapists use the teachings in the scriptures as a basis on which to assess their clients' psychological conditions, then based upon the assessments, decide the content of yoga therapy instruction for the clients.

Verse 4:*Hypocrisy, arrogance, self-conceit, harshness and also anger and ignorance, belong to one who is born in a demoniacal state, O Arjuna!*

Yoga Therapy Theory

Verse 5:*The divine nature is deemed for liberation and the demoniacal for bondage. Grieve not, O Arjuna, for thou art born with divine properties!*

Commentary: In this stressful modern society, we are attached to many things, and these attachments create disturbances in our minds. There is a need to both prevent and heal many psychosomatic and lifestyle diseases. How should we handle these external stressors, and how can we maintain our mental and physical condition? One solution is written in this verse. If we cultivate our divine qualities, if we cultivate healthy qualities that lead to healthy psychological responses, we can liberate ourselves from stressors. Yoga therapy techniques help people heal themselves, and cultivating these healthy qualities is what yoga therapy is about. Yoga therapists also help clients to let go of unhealthy responses and develop healthy psychological responses by using relevant teachings in the scriptures to provide psychoeducation for the client.

Verse 21:*Triple is the gate of this hell, destructive of the self—lust, anger, and greed,—therefore, one should abandon these three.*
Verse 22: *A man who is liberated from these three gates to darkness, O Arjuna, practices what is good for him and thus goes to the Supreme goal!*
Verse 23:*He who, casting aside the ordinances of the scriptures, acts under the impulse of desire, attains neither perfection nor happiness nor the supreme goal.*
Verse 24:*Therefore, let the scripture be the authority in determining what ought to be done and what ought not to be done. Having known what is said in the ordinance of the scriptures, thou shouldst act here in this world.*

Commentary: This "gate of hell" described earlier is the same as the quality of tamas in Ayurveda. A tamas-predominant state is characterized by lust, anger, and greed. Professor Hiroshi Utena from Tokyo University Medical School's psychiatric department has often said that the most troublesome stressors for clients with schizophrenia are "relationships, money, and pride." This is probably true for most people, not only those with schizophrenia. People struggle with relationships, finances, anger, and self-esteem. It would thus be helpful for anyone to overcome these stressors by developing higher qualities in everyday life. This is precisely what yoga therapists teach, so it is important that yoga therapists assess the degree to which rajas and tamas are prevalent in their clients. After that, during counseling, the yoga therapist will become aware of the client's wrong cognition habits that lie behind his/her desire for affection, greed, and anger. After that, yoga therapists can help clients through psychoeducation to notice their own misunderstanding. Similar insights can also occur in meditation during yoga therapy instruction.

3) Yoga Therapy Assessment (YTA) and Ayurvedic Assessment

In the *Charaka Samhita*, there are assessment methods such as the ones introduced in the verses that follow. In yoga therapy, we also utilize Ayurvedic assessment methods to assess clients' mental states.

Charaka Samhita: Sharira Sthana **Chapter IV Verse 34**

> *There are three physical doshas (vitiating elements), viz., vata, pitta and kapha—they vitiate the body. Again there are two mental doshas, viz., rajas and tamas—they vitiate the mind. Vitiation of the body and the mind result in the manifestation of diseases—there is no disease without their vitiation.*

Commentary

There are doshas in both the body and the mind, and the mental doshas are tamas and rajas. These mental doshas are, to borrow

Yoga Therapy Theory

the expression from the *Bhagavad Gita*, "demonic qualities." It is necessary for the yoga therapist to assess the degree that these problematic qualities exist in the client.

Charaka Samhita: Vimanasthana Chapter VIII Verse 119

The patient is again to be examined with reference to his sattva *or mental faculties.* Sattva *is mind, and it regulates the body because of its association with the soul. Depending upon its strength, it is of three types, viz., superior, mediocre, and inferior. Thus human beings are classified into three categories depending upon the superiority, mediocrity, or inferiority of their mental faculties. Individuals having mental faculties of superior type are possessed of the excellence of these faculties, and the characteristic features of such individuals are described above. Even if possessed of weak physique, such individuals, because of the specific manifestations of* sattva *qualities in them, tolerate serious exogenous and endogenous diseases without much difficulty. Individuals having mediocrity of mental faculties tolerate the pain themselves when they realise that others can also tolerate it. Then they at times gain strength from others. Those having inferior type of mental faculties, neither by themselves nor through others can sustain their mental strength and even if possessed of plump or big physique, they cannot tolerate even mild pain. They are susceptible to fear, grief, greed, delusion and ego. When they hear even stories describing wrathful, fearful, hateful, terrifying and ugly situation or come across visions of flesh or blood of an animal or man they fall victims to depression, pallor, fainting, madness, giddiness of falling on the ground, or such events may even lead them to death.*

Commentary

In this verse, Charaka classifies the human psyche into three types according to strength—superior, medium, and inferior. This is the same as the categories of sattva (superior), rajas (medium), and tamas (inferior). Yoga instructors and yoga therapists should assess their client's mental condition and then provide instruction in yoga therapy accordingly.

4) Yoga Therapy Assessment (YTA) and Counseling Skills

It is very important that yoga therapists acquire skills in counseling in order to conduct effective yoga therapy assessments on the basis of the human structure and function theories introduced here and to design the best yoga therapy practices for their clients. Considering the numbers of people with psychosomatic ailments coming to yoga classes all over the world, yoga instructors should also assess the mental and physical conditions of their clients and students that they meet for the first time.

Listed subsequently are areas that all yoga therapists should study in order to develop their skills to be effective counselors.

i) The need for counseling skills
ii) Counseling techniques for accurate YTA
  a. Intake interview skills
  b. Practices for collecting information
  c. YTI contract

I strongly encourage yoga instructors who sincerely strive to support their students to acquire this type of expertise and develop as professionals.

PART III

The Koshas: Yoga Therapy Assessment (YTA) and Yoga Therapy Instruction (YTI)

CHAPTER 1

Yoga Therapy Assessment (YTA) and Yoga Therapy Instruction (YTI) for the Annamaya Kosha

1) Yoga Therapy's Pathogenesis Theory and the Annamaya Kosha

In conventional medicine, diseases are considered to be caused by pathogens or physical malfunctions. In the case of yoga therapy (which is also a way to implement Ayurvedic psychological and spiritual treatments), the first stage of illnesses is when afflicted memories (memories causing suffering) disrupt the normal functioning of the buddhi, the psychological organ of the vijnanamaya kosha. This leads to predominance in mental doshas (i.e., mental disturbance), eventually disrupting the functions of the manomaya and pranamaya koshas, and finally leading to malfunctions in the annamaya kosha, the physical body.

Conventional medicine's approach to disease is generally limited to this last annamaya kosha stage. According to yoga therapy, the buddhi's job is to recognize, discern, predict, decide, and issue executive orders for action through the manas (psychological organ of the manomaya kosha). It is, therefore, important to ensure that no problems arise in the transfer of information between the buddhi and manas. Using the human chariot theory, if the ten horses (organs of perception and action) function in an unhealthy manner, the brain—part of the annamaya kosha—is affected, and disrupted brain functioning creates disturbance in breathing, which is regulated by the central nervous system. The endocrine system and immune system may also be disrupted, and this leads to various kinds of disorders in the organs, as well as in motor, intellectual and mental capacity.

In this way, psychological disorders due to stress, such as psychosomatic disorders, lifestyle diseases, and mental illness, have their root causes in poor functioning of the buddhi, the impacts of which eventually manifest in the annamaya kosha as physical disorders. I will explain more about the functions of the vijnanamaya kosha in chapter IV. In this chapter, I will explain in particular about how yoga therapy can address physical problems (annamaya kosha) that have their roots in the vijnanamaya kosha.

2) Yoga Therapy Assessment (YTA) of the Annamaya Kosha

A. Assessing Physical Functions (Alexisomia[35])

The disorders and diseases of the physical body that yoga therapy addresses are psychosomatic disorders, such as the ones listed subsequently. Yoga therapists should take into consideration any diagnoses from medical doctors, ask clients about symptoms, assess the clients' range of motion, pain, and other physical conditions, and then after that, assess how the vijnanamaya kosha is responsible for these problems. This assessment is unique to yoga therapy. To conduct these assessments, we have developed YTA tools based on Ayurveda and traditional yoga's theory of humans functions. After the initial assessment is complete, clients begin a yoga therapy practice using yoga therapy techniques for the annamaya kosha. Following is a list of medical conditions that medical doctors have also begun attributing at least partially to psychological factors.

---

35 Alexisomia is the English term for "shitsu-taikan-sho" in Japanese. It was coined in 1979 by Dr. Yujiro Ikemi, and is defined as "the condition of having difficulty in experiencing bodily feelings (shitsu=lack, taikan=bodily feelings, sho=symptoms or conditions." http://okat.web.fc2.com/page02_03_2.html. Accessed August 24, 2016.

Yoga Therapy Theory

B. Examples of Medical Conditions Caused by Disrupted Mental Functions (Psychosomatic Illness)

- *Circulatory system*: high blood pressure, ischemic heart disease (coronary infarction, angina pectoris)
- *Digestive system*: peptic ulcer (stomach, duodenum, bowels) irritable bowel syndrome
- *Respiratory system*: bronchial asthma, hyperventilation syndrome
- *Metabolic system*: diabetes, hyperthyroid
- *Neuro/Muscular system*: migraine, torticollis, tic
- *Skin disease*: atopic dermatitis, alopecia areata
- *Orthopedics*: rheumatoid arthritis, lower back pain, fibromyalgia
- *Urology*: bed-wetting, enuresis, frequent urination
- *Gynecology*: menopausal disorder, menstrual pain, irregular menstruation
- *Pediatrics*: bronchial asthma, irritable bowel syndrome, anorexia nervosa
- *Ear, nose, and throat*: Meniere's disease, nasal allergy, stammering
- *Oral/Dental*: temporomandibular dysfunction syndrome, trigeminal neuralgia

C. Examples of Psychological Disorders That Can Arise from Disrupted Mental Functions

- Panic disorder
- Bipolar disorder
- Eating disorder
- Personality disorder
- Sleeping disorder
- Posttraumatic stress disorder (PTSD)

People with illnesses in acute stages generally do not go to ordinary yoga studios. We are seeing, however, people recently released from hospitals or undergoing outpatient treatment increasingly turning to yoga in the hope of preventing recurrence of their illness and wanting to build both mental and physical strength. Though yoga studios are not medical facilities, people whose illnesses are in remission or people who have chronic illnesses also go to yoga classes. There is a growing need for capacity building and education to increase the numbers of yoga therapists who are capable of working with medical professionals. Considering this trend, it is of utmost importance that yoga instructors are also trained in basic yoga therapy and know how to refer people with illnesses to yoga therapists possessing the necessary expertise.

3) Ayurveda-Based Yoga Therapy Assessment

A. Prakrti—Psychosomatic Constitution

When people who have been diagnosed with illnesses by medical doctors come to yoga studios hoping to maintain their recently recovered health, one YTA tool that can be used examines the individual's *prakrti*, or psychosomatic constitution according to Ayurveda. A person's prakrti is determined at birth and does not change over time, so it continues to affect the person throughout their entire life.

There is currently research being supported by the Indian government that is examining the relationship between prakrti and genes, and researchers are finding that they do indeed coincide.[36] Knowing one's prakrti can be very helpful for living a long, healthy life. Various factors determine one's prakrti, and in Ayurveda, there are seven different types. They are (1) vata, (2) pitta, (3) kapha, (4) vata-pitta, (5) pitta-kapha, (6)

---

36 R. C. Juyal, S. Negi, P. Wakhode, et al. "Potential of Ayurgenomics Approach in Complex Trait Research: Leads from a Pilot Study on Rheumatoid Arthritis," PLoS ONE 7, no. 9 (2012): e45752, doi: 10.1371/journal.pone.0045752.

kapha-vata, and (7) vata-pitta-kapha. The three types of mental tempera-ments are (1) sattva, (2) rajas, and (3) tamas. If you are interested to know your prakrti, you can consult a certified yoga therapist or an Ayurvedic doctor. Following is a chart that can be used as an initial self-evaluation checklist to help you get an idea of which doshas are most predominant in your constitution.

B. Dosha Self-Evaluation Charts

Dr. Kazuo Uebaba created and published the following chart to do a self-evaluation of prakrti.[37] With the author's permission, we have included the chart that follows. The second self-evaluation chart following it measures vikrti, the current degree of imbalance of the doshas.

* ***Dosha* Self-Evaluation Chart**
   Circle the degree to which each sentence has applied to you since childhood, then calculate your innate constitution.

   Keep the right VPK columns hidden from view as you circle the number that is most applicable to each sentence. After cir-cling a number, write that number in the open box to the right (under V, P, or K). After completing all the questions, total the numbers for each dosha. Your prakrti is the ratio indicated by each dosha score.

---

37 Kazuo Uebaba. *Yasashii Ayurveda* ("Easy Ayurveda" in Japanese). PHP Institute, Tokyo, 1996.

Prakrti (innate constitution) Assessment Chart Circle the number that most accurately applies to you since childhood.	Never	Rarely	Some-times	Usually	Always	V	P	K
I am a perfectionist, and I also hold others to high standards.	1	2	3	4	5	■		■
I dislike cold and wet climates, and easily get a runny nose.	1	2	3	4	5	■		■
I adapt to new environments with great ease.	1	2	3	4	5	■		■
I have many freckles or moles on my skin.	1	2	3	4	5	■		■
I have strong interest in food, and spend a lot of money on meals.	1	2	3	4	5	■		■
My skin easily becomes flakey, especially in winter.	1	2	3	4	5	■		■
I learn new things quickly, but also forget quickly.	1	2	3	4	5	■		■
My body is warm and I sweat and become thirsty easily.	1	2	3	4	5		■	
I have a large body frame and my arms are strong.	1	2	3	4	5			■
I sunburn easily.	1	2	3	4	5		■	
I am reserved and shy.	1	2	3	4	5	■		
I often get heartburn and canker sores.	1	2	3	4	5		■	
My teeth are large and white, and I have few cavities.	1	2	3	4	5			■
I often feel bloated and pass gas frequently.	1	2	3	4	5	■		
I earn money quickly and spend it quickly too.	1	2	3	4	5	■		
My eyes tend to get bloodshot	1	2	3	4	5		■	
It takes me time to memorize something, but once I do, I do not forget.	1	2	3	4	5			■
My teeth are of various sizes and are crooked.	1	2	3	4	5	■		
I gain weight easily, and the blood vessels in my arms and legs are not easily visible.	1	2	3	4	5			■
I am very curious and interested in many things, but I do not stick with one thing for very long.	1	2	3	4	5	■		
I am a big eater and become irritable when I am hungry.	1	2	3	4	5		■	
Missing a meal does not bother me much.	1	2	3	4	5			■
I have a slender physique, or was initially slender.	1	2	3	4	5	■		
I am short tempered and get irritable or angry easily.	1	2	3	4	5		■	
My hair is dark, and my hair is thick for my age.	1	2	3	4	5			■
The blood vessels on my hands and feet protrude and are easy to see.	1	2	3	4	5	■		
I am concise in speech and action, and people say I am eloquent.	1	2	3	4	5		■	
I can sleep anywhere, and I am not lacking in sleep.	1	2	3	4	5			■
I tend to get constipated, especially if I skip breakfast.	1	2	3	4	5	■		
I am prematurely grey, and had early hair loss and/or premature wrinkles.	1	2	3	4	5		■	
My skin is soft and smooth, and I have a light complexion.	1	2	3	4	5			■
When I have to decide something, I tend to brood or debate and have difficulty deciding.	1	2	3	4	5	■		
My movements are fast and I tend to walk more quickly than people around me.	1	2	3	4	5	■		
I assert myself, am intellectual, smart, and am a good leader.	1	2	3	4	5		■	
I am calm and rarely get angry.	1	2	3	4	5			■
My face and skin tends to be reddish or yellowish.	1	2	3	4	5		■	
I can withstand vigorous exercise or physical labor.	1	2	3	4	5			■
I am sensitive to cold, and my hands and feet are cold.	1	2	3	4	5	■		
I pass stool at least once or more a day, and my stool is often very soft.	1	2	3	4	5			■
I am slow at walking or eating.	1	2	3	4	5			■
I move my hands and feet even when I am sitting.	1	2	3	4	5	■		
I like cold drinks and cold food.	1	2	3	4	5		■	
I rarely get irritated and I concentrate well.	1	2	3	4	5	■		■
My joints often make popping noises.	1	2	3	4	5	■		
I have intelligent and piercing eyes.	1	2	3	4	5		■	
						V	P	K
Total Points								
Ratio= Each dosha score/(V+P+K)								

Yoga Therapy Theory

Ayurveda explains that in order to live a healthy life, it helps to have a lifestyle that matches your prakrti, your inherent constitution. As you go about your daily life, weaknesses in your constitution can be affected by surrounding conditions, creating changes in the balance of your doshas. This is called vikrti, or your psychosomatic condition. You can check your current vikrti with the chart that follows. Answer the questions regarding your condition over the past week and see if there has been an increase or decrease in the doshas. You can also reflect upon what lifestyle influences may be at play in creating these changes.

* **Dosha Balance Self-Assessment Chart**

Questions for an Ayurvedic assessment of the degree of imbalance (vikrti) in your natural constitution.

Keeping the right side of the chart (VPK) hidden, circle the number that most accurately applies to your condition over the past week or so. After you are done, write the number you circled in the blank space to the right (under V, P, or K). When complete, total the scores for the three doshas.

Vikrti (dosha imbalance) Self-Assessment Chart Circle the number most applicable to your condition over the past week.	Never	Rarely	Some-times	Usually	Always	V	P	K
My skin is dry.	1	2	3	4	5		■	
The whites of my eyes are reddish and often bloodshot.	1	2	3	4	5	■		
Many thoughts come to mind, but I do not concentrate well.	1	2	3	4	5		■	
I eat a lot and until I am full.	1	2	3	4	5	■		
I often feel anxious and worry a lot.	1	2	3	4	5	■		
I am often thirsty.	1	2	3	4	5		■	
My stool is often loose and I get diarrhea easily.	1	2	3	4	5		■	
It takes a long time to fall asleep, and I am a light sleeper.	1	2	3	4	5	■		
I doze off quickly and am often drowsy.	1	2	3	4	5	■		■
I get red rashes on my skin.	1	2	3	4	5	■	■	
I smoke or drink alcohol a lot.	1	2	3	4	5	■		
I often feel unwell in cold and wet weather.	1	2	3	4	5			■
I have phlegm and cough a lot.	1	2	3	4	5			■
I often feel wide awake and cannot sleep.	1	2	3	4	5		■	
I have a lot of gas and flatulence.	1	2	3	4	5	■		
I tend to be constipated.	1	2	3	4	5	■		
My arms and legs tend to feel heavy; my joints hurt.	1	2	3	4	5	■		
I easily get welt-like rashes.	1	2	3	4	5		■	
My face or nose is reddish.	1	2	3	4	5		■	
I am short-tempered and irritable, and am quick to see other people's faults.	1	2	3	4	5		■	
My body feels heavy, and it is a lot of trouble to do anything.	1	2	3	4	5			■
I often want cold drinks or cold food.	1	2	3	4	5		■	
I get canker sores, or my mouth feels sticky.	1	2	3	4	5			■
I tire easily and feel dispirited by afternoon.	1	2	3	4	5	■		
The inside of my mouth is sweet. Or the inside of my mouth feels sticky.	1	2	3	4	5			■
It does not bother me to skip meals.	1	2	3	4	5	■		
I am unmotivated and back away from doing things.	1	2	3	4	5			■
I sleep solidly for at least 8 hours.	1	2	3	4	5			■
I sweat a lot.	1	2	3	4	5		■	
I get heartburn or burning sensations in my anus.	1	2	3	4	5		■	
I am a light sleeper and have scary or anxious dreams.	1	2	3	4	5	■		
My heart pounds for no particular reason.	1	2	3	4	5	■		
I catch colds easily and usually have a runny or congested nose.	1	2	3	4	5			■
My hands and feet are cold, and I feel cold easily.	1	2	3	4	5	■		
I feel pain such as headaches, stomach aches, muscle pain, or cramps/twitches.	1	2	3	4	5	■		
I feel lethargic and unmotivated in the mornings.	1	2	3	4	5			■
						V	P	K
				Total points				

Yoga Therapy Theory

By understanding our prakrti and regularly checking our vikrti, we learn to assess our annamaya kosha in accordance with Ayurvedic principles. I hope that Dr. Uebaba's assessment tools are useful for you to develop the habit of checking your physical condition and integrating this kind of wisdom into your daily life by deepening your understanding of the doshas.

4) Principles of Yoga Therapy Instruction (YTI) for the Annamaya Kosha

The aim of these yoga therapy practices for the annamaya kosha is actually to develop the ability to observe and be aware of changes that occur in the body during and after the practices. This is basic practice in self-control, and for clients with psychosomatic or lifestyle diseases, self-control is a key factor in reclaiming health. Developing self-mastery is helpful not only in yoga therapy, but in traditional Raja Yoga, self-control is said to be the way to unite with the true Self.

> "The *Yoga Sutras* of Patanjali consider every kind of self, every stage of self, which has to be subdued in the process called self-control—reaching, finally, the control the whole Self, which is universally spread out. From the stage of the lower conception of the self, which is to be restrained in self-control, we reach a higher Self, which is realized simultaneously. Therefore, self-restraint and Self-realization are simultaneous things; they mean one and the same thing." (*The Epistemology of Yoga* by Swami Krishnananda)[38]

Swami Krishnananda was the secretary-general of the Shivananda Yoga Ashram in Muni Ki Reti, Rishikesh, Uttarakhand, India. I met him many times when I went to his office to organize a Japanese translation of his book, and I was always very impressed by his intelligence. He

---

38 Swami Krishnananda, The Epistemology of Yoga, (Rishikesh, India: The Divine Life Society, Sivananda Ashram), e-book edition.

could explain difficult yogic concepts in simple words, as in this quote above. These principles of self-control that lead us to truth can be applied to the methods of yoga therapy instruction that I am explaining in this book. Now I will explain some of these teaching methods and practices.

A. Yoga Therapy Techniques and Principles of Practice for the Annamaya Kosha

Unlike traditional yoga, the instruction and practice of yoga therapy is for the general public, and in particular, people with various disorders or illnesses. The results of our survey on adverse events in yoga that I introduced at the beginning of this book made it clear that teaching yoga to general populations without assessing students is potentially dangerous, and this is why it is necessary to be aware of individual health conditions and to adapt traditional practices to suit their conditions. Aside from meditation and pranayama practices, yoga therapy techniques for the annamaya kosha can be divided roughly into the categories explained subsequently. All of them incorporate the principles of the traditional discipline of yoga, that is, strength building and mental training, which develops awareness of oneself here and now.

1) Breathing exercises (with or without isometric resistance, slow training)
2) Sukshma vyayama, (with or without isometric resistance, slow training)
3) Asana (with or without isometric breathing, slow training)

Each of these yoga therapy technique categories contains several types of exercises, and a few will be introduced with photos that follow. These techniques are being used by yoga therapists throughout Japan. Since 2009, JYTS has also been teaching these techniques to people who were exposed to radiation from the Chernobyl nuclear accident. We are

Yoga Therapy Theory

working with teachers and medical professionals in Kiev and are seeing outstanding results, including normalization of blood pressure and oxidative stress levels.

We have been teaching the two following yoga therapy programs in Kiev. We made a DVD of these programs in Japanese, and after northeast Japan was hit by the earthquake, tsunami and nuclear accident in Fukushima in March 2011, we made thirty thousand copies and distributed them free of charge in affected areas. In July 2014, we made a second yoga therapy program DVD, also for people still affected by the 2011 disaster, and are introducing the program in this book. We use this as a charity initiative as well. A purchase of one DVD for two thousand yen (approximately 20 US dollars) enables us to make ten DVDs for free distribution in northeastern Japan, or for people who had to evacuate their homes and are currently living in other parts of the country.

Each program that follows lasts approximately twenty minutes. Simple movements are coordinated with breathing, and isometric resistance is used with chanting the n-kara (or "n-sound"). The n-kara can be done aloud or mentally. All isometric resistance should use only half or one-third of your full strength. Exerting too much effort can increase blood pressure, so elderly and people with hypertension should be particularly careful.

YOGA FOR ANTI-AGEING: SEATED PROGRAM (20 MINUTES)

In this seated program, begin each posture with your palms resting on your thighs. When you complete the given number of rounds, make sure to take time to sit and observe your natural breathing.

A similar program can also be viewed online at this URL: https://youtu.be/s-lt9M_k2Do

1. Natural Breath Observation (for 1 minute with eyes closed)
Sit comfortably. Place your palms on your abdomen, and feel how the abdomen moves with the breath.

2. Arms Behind the Back Pose: Five rounds

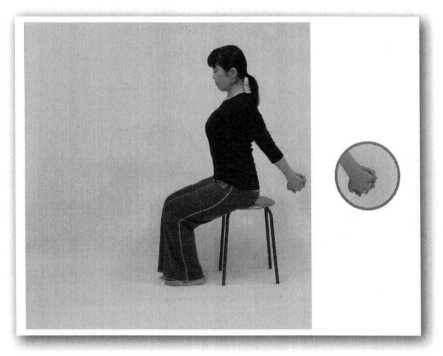

Begin seated with your palms resting on your thighs.

As you inhale, bring both arms behind your back, interlock your fingers, and expand the chest. As you exhale, say, "nnn" (aloud or mentally) and grip the hands and tighten the arms and shoulders. Inhale and release the tension in the shoulders, arms, and hands. Exhale saying, "nnn" (aloud or mentally) as you return your hands to the top of the thighs. After completing five rounds, rest and observe your natural breath.

3. Palm of the Hand Press: Five rounds

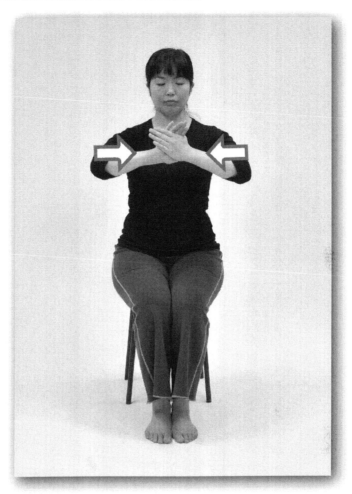

Begin by sitting with your palms resting on your thighs.

As you inhale, bring the palms of the hands diagonally together in front of the chest. Exhale while saying, "nnn" (aloud or mentally) and press the palms together, feeling how the body tenses. Inhale and release the pressure of the hands. Then exhale with the sound, "nnn" (aloud or mentally) as you return your palms to the top of the thighs. When you have finished, rest and observe your natural breath.

4. Palm of the Hand Pulling: Five rounds

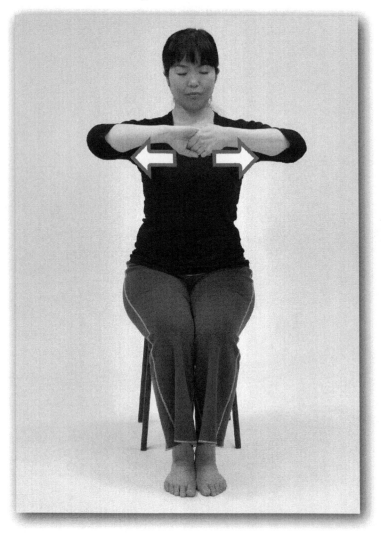

As you inhale, raise the hands to chest level and join the palms in a diagonal handshake. Exhale and say, "nnn" (aloud or mentally) while pulling the hands in opposite directions. Inhale and release all the tension, then exhale and say, "nnn" (aloud or mentally) as you return both palms on top of the thighs. When you have finished, rest and observe your natural breath.

5. Front and Back Ankle Push: Three rounds

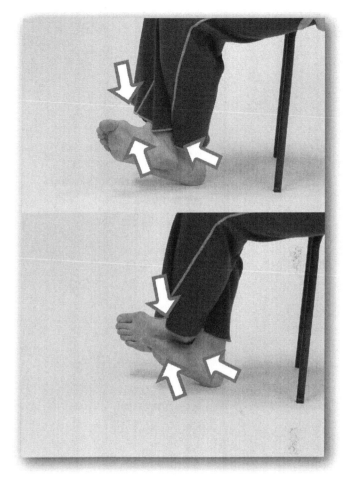

Sit with the soles of both feet flat on the floor.

As you inhale, cross your ankles. Keep the heel of the back foot on the floor. Exhale while saying, "nnn" (aloud or mentally), and press the ankles against each other (in a forward and back direction). Inhale to release the pressure, then exhale saying, "nnn" (aloud or mentally) as you uncross the ankles and return both feet to the floor. Then as you inhale, repeat the same but with the opposite foot in front. This is one round. When you have finished, rest and observe your natural breath.

6. Outside Knee Push: Five rounds

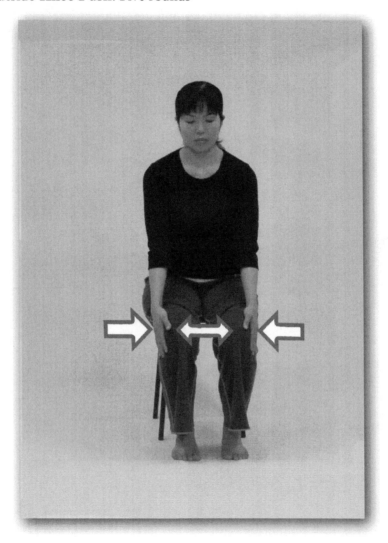

As you inhale, place your palms on the outside of your knees. As you exhale, say, "nnn" (aloud or mentally), pressing the knees outward and resisting the palms inward. Release the pressure as you inhale, then exhale again saying, "nnn" (aloud or mentally) as you return your palms to your thighs. When you have finished, rest and observe your natural breath.

7. Twist Pose: Three rounds

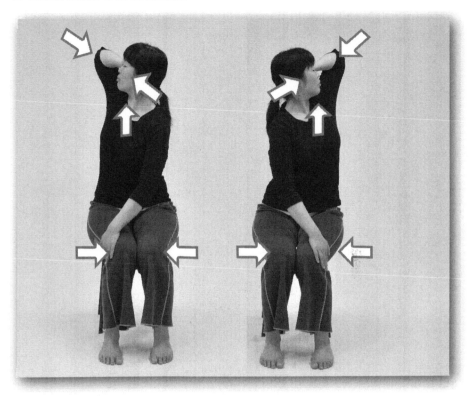

Begin seated with both hands on your thighs.

As you inhale, bring your left hand to the outside of your right knee. Also bring your right palm to the right side of your head. As you exhale saying, "nnn" (aloud or mentally), press the hand and knee, and the hand and head against each other. As you inhale, release the pressure, and then exhale saying, "nnn," and return both palms to rest on the thighs. Then repeat the same on the other side to complete one round. When you have finished, rest and observe your natural breath.

8. Easy Abdominal Breathing (Sukha Pranayama): 1 minute with eyes closed

Sit comfortably. Inhale easily, then exhale for twice the length of the inhalation. Practice breathing with awareness and with a one-to-two ratio of inhalation to exhalation.

When you have finished, slowly transition into your daily activities.

YOGA FOR ANTI-AGEING: STANDING PROGRAM (20 MINUTES)

Available online at: www.youtube.com/watch?v=_19PR8esA34
*After completing each exercise, rest and observe the natural breath for about five to ten breaths before beginning the next exercise.

1. Breath Awareness: 1 minute with eyes closed

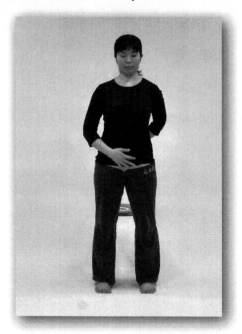

Place one hand on your abdomen and one on your lower back. Feel how your body moves as you breathe.

Yoga Therapy Theory

2. Both Arms Behind the Back Stretch: Five rounds

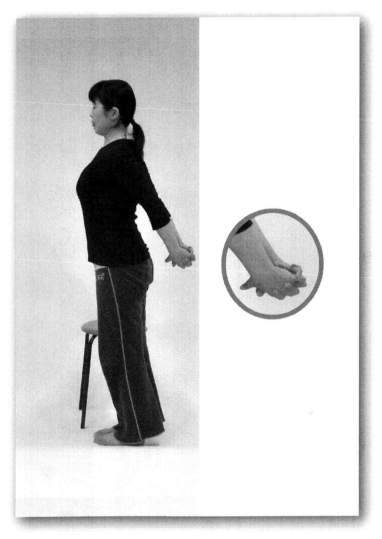

As you inhale, bring both arms behind your back and interlock your fingers. As you exhale, say, "nnn" (aloud or mentally) while gripping the hands, tensing the arms and shoulders, and broadening the chest. As you inhale, release the tension, and then exhale saying, "nnn" (aloud or mentally) as you return your arms to relax at your sides.

3. Lower Back Pushing: Five rounds

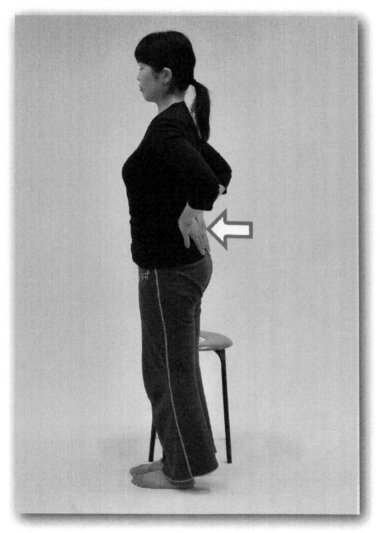

As you inhale, place the palms of both hands on your lower back and expand the chest fully. Exhale saying, "nnn" (aloud or mentally) as you press the palms and your lower back against each other. Inhale and release the pressure. Exhale saying, "nnn" (aloud or mentally) as you lower your arms to your sides.

4. Standing Twist Pose: Three rounds

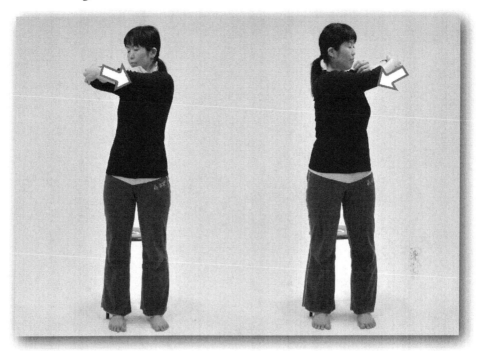

As you inhale, bring your left hand to the outside of your right elbow, while turning your head and torso about forty-five degrees to the right. Then as you exhale, say "nnn" (aloud or mentally) and create isometric resistance with the elbow and hand. Inhale to return to face forward and once again say, "nnn" (aloud or mentally) as you release the hands down to your sides. Repeat the same on the other side. Once on each side is one round.

5. Knee Push: Three rounds

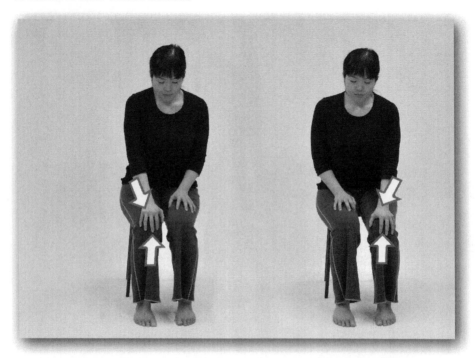

Sit in a chair. As you exhale saying, "nnn" (aloud or mentally), lift your leg up as you press down with the palm of your hand. Inhale once, and then exhale saying, "nnn" (aloud or mentally), releasing the pressure. Repeat the same with the opposite leg and hand. This is one round.

6. Inward Knee Press: Three rounds

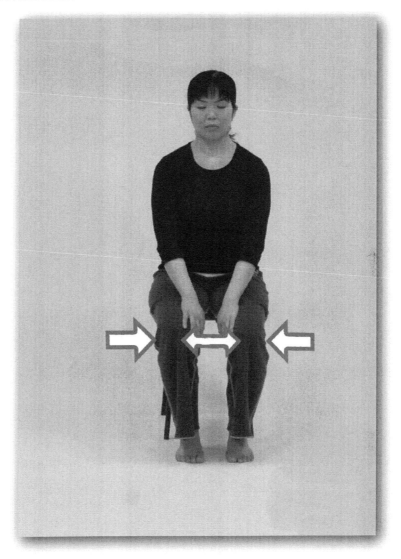

As you inhale, bring your palms to the inside of each knee. Exhale saying, "nnn" (aloud or mentally) while pressing the palms and knees against each other. As you inhale, release the pressure, then again exhale saying, "nnn" (aloud or mentally) and bring the palms to the tops of the thighs.

7. Agni Prasarana (Bellow Breathing): Ten repetitions/Fifteen repetitions

Agni prasarana uses the abdomen to create strong inhalations and exhalations, at the pace of about one breath per second. In a seated posture, do one set of ten repetitions. Rest for a while, then do another set of fifteen repetitions.

*When you have completed the whole program, slowly return to your daily activities.

A similar program can also be viewed online at <https://youtu.be/_l9PR8esA34>. If you are interested to practice along with a DVD, we have made one in English, and it can be ordered from the Japan Yoga Therapy Society.

In the following reference, I will introduce some teachings from the ancient scriptures. They will help to better understand the significance of traditional yoga practices.

———

REFERENCE 2: RAJA YOGA TEXT

Patanjali's *Yoga Sutras* Chapter 2 Verse 46

Posture (should be) steady and comfortable.

Commentary: This is Patanjali's definition of asana. Traditionally, yogis traveled to the Himalayas and stayed in areas where very few people visited, much less lived. My guru, Swami Yogeshwarananda, was also a traditional Raja Yogi. When he lived in the Himalayas, he walked where there were no roads, climbed rocks with bare hands, and crossed rivers where there were no bridges. His asana instruction was clearly to build the physical strength and endurance to survive rugged and harsh Himalayan conditions. He did not teach his disciples how to strike beautiful poses or consider asana to be exercise. In fact, he reprimanded people who practiced in this way, challenging them to consider the purpose of their asana practice. Focusing a yoga practice on how to do poses was, in his words, "acrobatics and childish play."

Repeatedly stretching muscles weakens them, and would make it impossible for yogis to survive the traditional and harsh training in the Himalayas. It is safe to say that practice of modern acrobatic poses (which may seem similar to traditional postures but are worlds apart) cannot develop the physique and mental toughness attained by traditional yogis. The purpose of traditional asanas is to strengthen both the physical body and mind to enable sitting in meditation for hours at a time. With this, it becomes possible to sit comfortably and liberate ourselves from many stresses.

The yoga therapy practices that I introduce in this chapter are based on traditional asana. The techniques are adapted into exercises that anyone can do, but the principles and essence of traditional yoga are maintained. Also, scientific research on these yoga therapy practices utilizing isometric resistance is showing that they are inducing anti-ageing physiological responses, such as increases in growth hormones. This is not only about muscles; research in the field of neurosurgery shows that these exercises also help cranial nerves rejuvenate in people with dementia.[39] It is desirable that yoga instruction and practice is done with this understanding of such physiological mechanisms.

Yoga Sutras Chapter 2 Verse 47

By relaxation of effort and meditation on the "Endless" (posture is mastered).

Commentary: The purpose of asana is to enable us to sit for extended periods of time in meditation. Meditation techniques practiced in traditional yoga were for mental and spiritual training, so as yoga practice

---

39 Matsumi Seki et al., "Effect of Yoga therapy in day care for the patient in early stage of dementia," *The Journal of Japan Society for Early Stage of Dementia* 8, no. 2 (2015): 93.

advances, it becomes increasingly unnecessary to turn attention to the physical body. If the body gets tired easily sitting in a meditative posture, or if the muscles get too tense and start to hurt, such physical sensations disturb mental concentration. If you have any experience sitting in meditation or at a Zen temple and felt pain in your legs, you know very well how easy it is to be distracted by the body. On the other hand, when we are able to sit relaxed for extended periods of time without having to pay attention to the body, our minds and awareness naturally begin to turn to "the Endless" to eventually be absorbed. For this purpose, it is important to prepare the body and develop both physical and mental strength. This is also the purpose of the physical practices in yoga therapy.

Yoga Sutras Chapter 2 Verse 48

From that (mastery of posture) no assaults from the pairs of opposites.

Commentary: When practicing yoga therapy's physical techniques, people find that they are less disturbed in their daily lives. This is because yoga therapy is instructed in a way to ensure that practitioners remain focused on the changes happening here and now in their bodies. This is a practice in pulling away from the "pairs of opposites," or the duality that ordinarily creates stress and confusion in our daily lives, such as like/dislike, loss/gain, success/failure, friend/foe, good/bad, and so on. This is why Patanjali says that asana practice helps us to overcome duality. We can say that traditional yoga and even yoga therapy practices are psychotherapy, and in particular, traditional yoga practice enables the yogi to achieve a state that transcends duality through asana practice. Such training is useful for those who suffer psychosomatic illnesses, as it helps them overcome over-adaptive tendencies. Over-adaptation is common among people with psychosomatic disorders. It is a tendency to pay too much attention to what is happening outside of oneself. Many people with psychosomatic disorders who are practicing yoga therapy are enjoying many

Yoga Therapy Theory

improvements to their health. We collect case studies every year. If you are interested in seeing information on case studies, please contact the Japan Yoga Therapy Society.

Yoga Sutras Chapter 2 Verse 49

This having been (accomplished), pranayama, which is cessation of inspiration and expiration (follows).

Commentary: In the eight limbs of yoga, pranayama follows asana. This is because pranayama deals with a realm subtler than the physical body. While doing asanas primarily involves the muscles, pranayama controls the breath and is related to the autonomic nervous system. The breath is also said to be the bridge between body and mind. In yoga therapy, controlling the inhalation and exhalation is not only exercising control over our autonomic nervous system, it also impacts our endocrine and immune systems, which are deeply related to the autonomic nervous system. We are seeing how effective pranayama can be in restoring the health of people with imbalance in the relationship between body and mind when the program is based on a thorough yoga therapy assessment. Pranayama is useful for promoting health in a dimension different than that treated by conventional medicine and surgery. Please see the following chapter on the pranamaya kosha to read about research that has been done on the physiological effects of pranayama.

REFERENCE 3: HATHA YOGA SCRIPTURE
From *Hatha Yoga Pradipika* of Maharaji Svatmarama

Chapter 1 on Asana, Verse 17

Prior to everything, asana is spoken of as the first part of Hatha Yoga. Having done asana one gets steadiness (firmness) of body and mind; diseaselessness and lightness (flexibility) of the limbs.

Commentary: The *Hatha Yoga Pradipika* is said to have been written in the fifteenth century, and the author says that one attains both physical and mental steadiness, good health, and a sense of lightness through the practice of Hatha Yoga, the physical discipline of traditional yoga. I think that the ancient yogis were well aware of this, and it is also experienced in yoga therapy practice. In modern society, the mechanism behind the effects of these practices is beginning to be understood in the medical and psychological fields. In the 1970s, I also went to the Himalayas and walked with yogis in places where there were no paths. There, I often saw yogis who wore only simple cloth shoes or even only rubber sandals, but who were able to walk like the wind through the mountains and over glaciers, and I believe this is what this verse is referring to. In yoga therapy, we maintain the essence, but modify the techniques so that anyone is able to practice. Without its essence, yoga's physical practices simply become "childish acrobatic play" to show off to others.

Chapter 1 Verse 67

Asanas, various types of kumbhaka, and the other various means of illumination should all be practiced in the Hatha Yoga system until success in Raja Yoga is attained.

Commentary: In this verse, the author of this scripture mentions asanas, kumbhaka, and mudras, and says that they are all basic practices of Raja Yoga. Raja Yoga is also known as *Ashtanga Yoga* (yoga of eight limbs), and the basic practices are classified into two kinds. One is the fundamental outer yoga (*bahiranga yoga*), which comprises the first five limbs of yama, niyama, asana, pranayama, and pratyahara. Then the second is the inner yoga, known as *antaranga yoga*, which is dharana, dhyana, and samadhi. This verse is referring to the inner yoga, and in yoga therapy, these inner yoga practices are known to have tremendous power in developing the ability to control body and mind.

Traditionally, special attention is given to the three limbs of inner yoga called *samyama*. Yoga therapists also use these three Raja Yoga methods to help clients transform the way they use their minds.

In India there is a saying that illustrates the understanding that mental conditions can affect one's entire life. They say, "when the mind changes, attitudes change. When attitudes change, behavior changes. When behavior changes, lifestyle changes. When lifestyle changes, personality changes. When personality changes, destiny changes."

I hope that readers of this book will begin yoga therapy practice, and find that it does indeed refine character and positively changes your destiny.

———

B. Yoga Therapy Instruction (YTI) for the Annamaya Kosha

Instruction of isometric breathing exercises, sukshma vyayama (with or without resistance/slow training) and asanas (with or without isometric resistance) for the annamaya kosha.

* Isometric breathing exercise practice
* Isometric sukshma vyayama practice

Next I will introduce some of the many techniques of the abovementioned practices. We have been distributing the following program free of charge to people affected by the 2011 eastern Japan earthquake and tsunami to promote their physical and mental health. If you would like more information, please contact us at JYTS.

ISOMETRIC YOGA THERAPY: SEATED PROGRAM

This program can also be viewed at this URL:
https://youtu.be/Ob7ZfQaQsmQ

(*All isometric pressure should be done gently, with only half or a third of your full strength.)

1. Natural Breath Awareness: Ten rounds

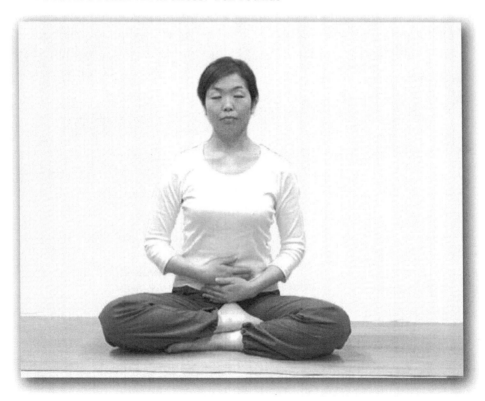

Place both palms on your abdomen and feel the movement of your natural breath. Count ten breaths.

2. **Seated Twisting**/right and left: Two rounds with or without n-kara.

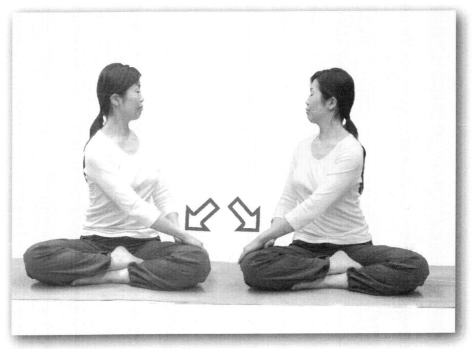

Begin in a neutral seated position. Then as you inhale, place both hands on the outside of your right (left) thigh. Press the hands and thigh against each other as you say, "nnn" (aloud or mentally). Do this twice. Then with an inhalation, release the pressure. Then exhale saying, "nnn," and return to the starting position.

3. **Seated Toe Pulling**/right and left: Two rounds with or without n-kara.

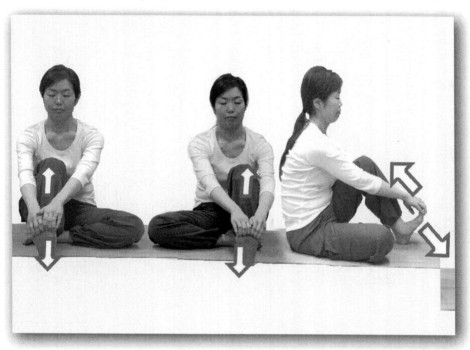

Hold your toes with both hands. As you say "nnn," use both hands to pull the toes of the right (left) foot, as you resist with the foot to press the toes down. Release the pressure as you inhale. Do this twice, and then return to the starting position as you exhale, saying, "nnn."

4. Seated Toe Pressing/ right and left: Two rounds with or without n-kara

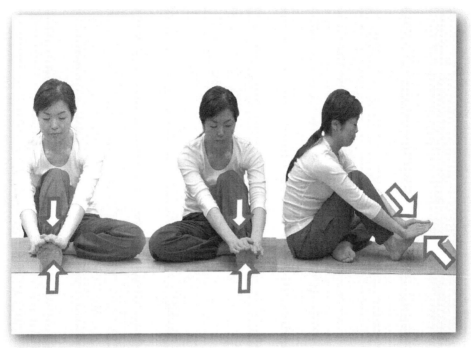

Bend your right (left) knee, and place both hands on top of your right (left) foot. As you press the top of the foot say, "nnn" and create isometric pressure. Release the pressure as you inhale. Do this twice, and then return to the starting position as you exhale, saying, "nnn."

5. Pressing Both Knees from Outside: Two rounds with or without n-kara

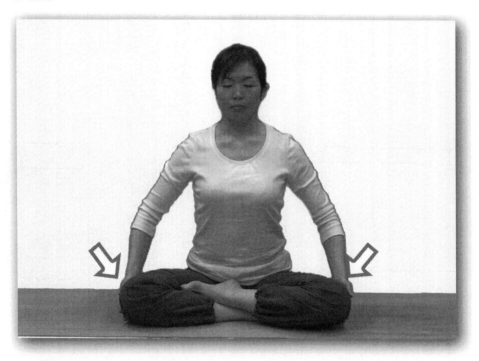

Inhale and place your palms on the outside of each knee. Exhale, saying, "nnn" and press the knees and palms against each other. Both hands should be pressing inward. Inhale and release the pressure. Do this twice, and then return to the starting position as you exhale, saying, "nnn."

6. Pulling Both Knees: Two rounds with or without n-kara.

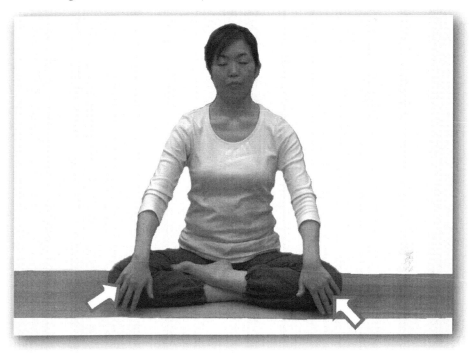

Inhale and place each palm on the front of each knee. Exhale, saying, "nnn," and use both hands to pull the knees so that the palm and knees are pushing against each other. Inhale releasing the pressure. Do this twice, and then return to the starting position as you exhale, saying, "nnn."

7. Lower Back Pressing: Two rounds with or without n-kara.

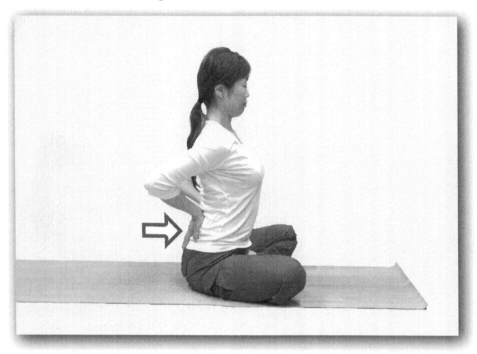

Place your palms on your lower back and as you say, "nnn," press your palms and lower back against each other. Inhale releasing the pressure. Do this twice, and then return to the starting position as you exhale, saying, "nnn."

8. Pressing the Back of the Head with the Palms: Two rounds with or without n-kara

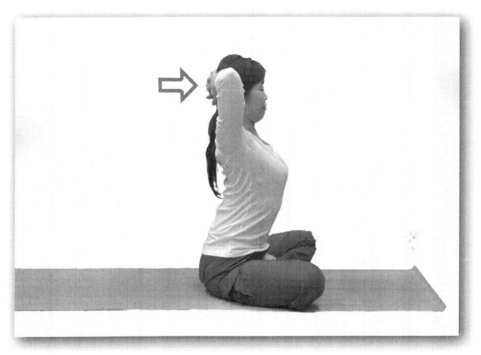

Bring the palms of both hands to the back of your head, and as you say, "nnn," press the palms and the back of your head against each other. Inhale releasing the pressure. Do this twice, and then return to the starting position as you exhale, saying, "nnn."

9. Shinkan (Mind Observation) Meditation: Two minutes

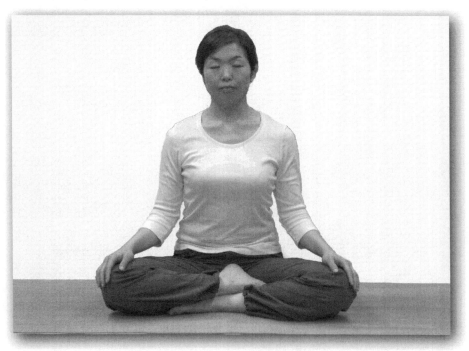

Close your eyes and just quietly observe as various thoughts and feelings arise and disappear. If a thought or feeling arises, then say to yourself, "I am thinking." When nothing arises, be aware of the absence of thought. This is a practice of the mind to simply watch the various thoughts that arise and disappear within it.

10. Abdominal breathing: Five rounds

Slowly inhale through the nose. Feel the abdomen expand. Say "nnn" as you exhale.

ISOMETRIC YOGA THERAPY: SUPINE PROGRAM

This program can also be viewed at this URL:
https://youtu.be/WlT3VdCBNMs

1. Breath Awareness: Ten natural abdominal breaths

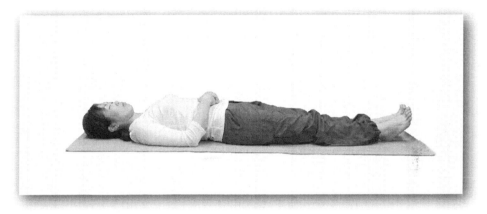

Place both palms on your abdomen and feel how the breath occurs naturally.

2. Supine Twisting/right and left: Two rounds with or without n-kara

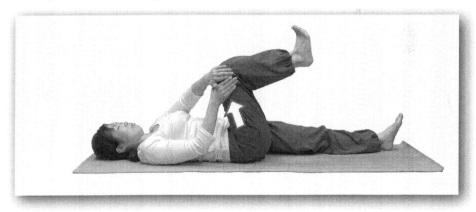

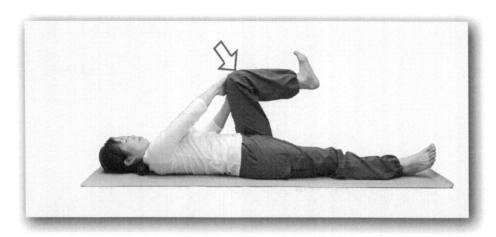

Bend the right (left) knee and raise it until you can touch it with both hands. Place both palms on the right (left) side of the right (left) knee. As you say "nnn," press the palms and the knee against each other. Inhale releasing the pressure. Exhale, saying, "nnn" and return to the starting position.

3. **Supine knee pressing**/right and left: Two rounds with or without n-kara

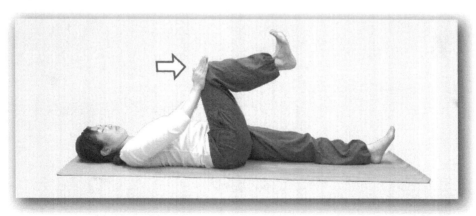

Bend your right (left) knee and raise it until you can reach it with both hands. Place both palms on the right (left) knee. Exhale, saying, "nnn" and press the palms and the knee against each other. Inhale releasing the pressure. Exhale, saying, "nnn" and return to the starting position.

4. Pressing Heels into Floor: Two rounds with or without n-kara

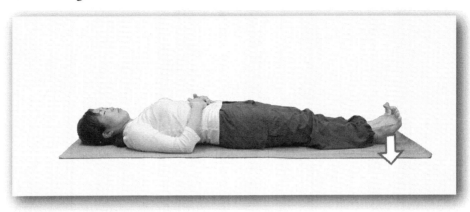

Spread your toes widely. As you say, "nnn" press your heels into the floor. Inhale and relax the toes and legs. Exhale, saying, "nnn" and allow the whole body to relax.

5. Pressing Elbows into the Floor: Two rounds with or without n-kara

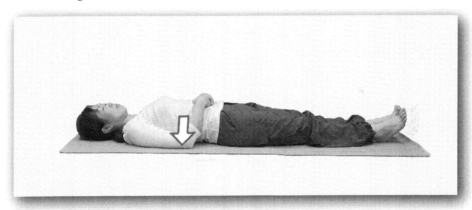

As you say, "nnn" press your elbows into the floor. Inhale and relax the arms. Exhale, saying, "nnn" and relax the entire body.

6. Supine Hip Raising: Two rounds with or without n-kara

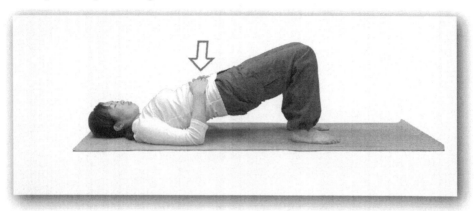

As you inhale slowly, bend both knees and lift your hips as high as you can, tightening the buttocks. Exhale, saying, "nnn," and release your hips to the floor.

7. Shinkan (Mind Observation) Meditation: Two minutes

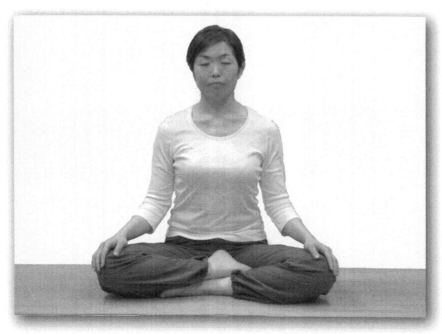

Close your eyes and just quietly observe as various thoughts and feelings arise and disappear. If a thought or feeling arises, say to yourself, "I am thinking." When nothing arises, be aware of the absence of thought. This is a practice of the mind to simply watch the various thoughts that arise and disappear within it.

8. Abdominal Breathing: Five rounds

Slowly inhale through the nose and feel the abdomen expand. Say, "nnn" as you exhale.

5) PREVENTION OF ADVERSE EVENTS IN THE ANNAMAYA KOSHA

Since 1987, JYTS has been cooperating with the headquarters of Swami Vivekananda Yoga Therapy Foundation/Yoga College, located in Bengaluru, Karnataka, India. As part of our work there, we have used breathing exercises that involve synchronizing movement of the body with breathing to help patients with psychosomatic and psychiatric disorders.

In these breathing exercises, we incorporate the use of sound. We generally use "ah," "oo," or "nnn," and these sounds can be vocalized aloud or done mentally. We also have two kinds of strength training, that is, isometric and isotonic training. Isometric exercises are stationary, and we call our isotonic exercises, "slow training," as it involves moving the body slowly while applying pressure. These techniques can be put into the following three categories:

- Breathing exercises without applying pressure
- Breathing exercises with isometric pressure
- Breathing exercises with slow training

Following is a list of precautions that practitioners and therapists should be aware of before doing these exercises.

1. **Degree of exerted strength:** Beginners should start with breathing exercises with slow training. These exercises have both movement

and applied pressure. It is easier for beginners to concentrate if there is some movement. It is important, however, to exercise caution in applying isometric or isotonic resistance. Pressing too hard can lead to adverse events, so make sure that you begin with an experienced instructor. Do not practice these carelessly on your own. In particular, it is difficult for elderly people to judge if they are using half, a third, a fourth, or maximum strength. Yoga therapists should consistently watch students to prevent accidents. If you are a beginner to this kind of yoga therapy, please find a certified therapist to instruct you.

2. **Be aware of changes between tension and relaxation:** In the case of breathing exercises or sukshma vyayama with slow training, it is quite easy to be aware of the difference between when muscles are tense and when they are relaxed, so it is a useful exercise to do on one's own at home.

3. **Progression in use of sounds:** When we do these exercises, yoga therapists generally use the sounds "ah," "oo," and "nnn." These three sounds can be used aloud or mentally. Start with "ah" and gradually introduce "oo." After this, "nnn" can be introduced. The sound "nnn" stimulates the olfactory nerve and other nerves in the nostrils, thus stimulating the entire brain. We call this "brain training." We are finding that this is very helpful for people with dementia.

4. **Notice changes in the length of exhalation:** Using the sounds "ah," "oo," and "nnn" aloud also facilitates lengthening the exhalation. "Nnn" generally naturally becomes the longest. This is said to stimulate the immune and endocrine systems and promote their healthy functioning.[40] Yoga therapists should explain this to their clients.

5. **Gradually increasing sensitivity to changes:** The difference between tension and relaxation is very easy to perceive in isometric

---

40 Tsutomu Kamei et. al., "Relationship between the Ratio of Change in Serum Cortisol and Change in Percent Alpha Time," *Perceptual and Motor Skills* 90 (2015): 1027–32.

slow training. Following that are practices using isometric pressure without movement, and then awareness with practices without isometric pressure. Yoga therapists should guide beginners with the techniques where change is easiest to feel, and progress to the subtler methods, thus developing more sensitivity to physical and physiological changes.

6. **Bringing internal changes into awareness with isometric pressure:** If you are new to these exercises, please receive instruction from a certified yoga therapist first. The yoga therapist will assess your physical and mental condition, and then introduce a program that will cultivate inner awareness through using the various isomeric exercises.

7. **In cases of sympathetic nervous system predominance:** When the sympathetic nervous system is predominant, it is recommended to begin with breathing exercises without isometric resistance that will help slow down the mind.

8. **Be aware of natural breathing after isometric practice:** After doing an isometric practice, spend some time observing the natural breath that occurs in the abdomen and/or chest. If you find it difficult to be aware of the breath, place your hands on your abdomen to make it easier to notice the movement of the body with the breath.

6) Fictional Case Studies: Annamaya Kosha

Every year, the Japan Yoga Therapy Society holds a research conference where yoga therapists present case studies of a format similar to the ones that follow. These case studies are contributing to a growing body of evidence for the effectiveness of yoga therapy. Following are two fictional case studies, the content of which comes from several actual cases. They have been compiled for educational purposes to show how yoga therapy can work for the annamaya kosha.

Kazuo Keishin Kimura

Fictional Case Study 1: Yoga Therapy for Rheumatoid Arthritis

1. Introduction

Rheumatoid arthritis is an immunological abnormality that affects various joints and causes edema and pain and sometimes destroys joints, changes their shape, and deprives them of movement. This is a case report in which a woman with rheumatoid arthritis was affected by stress due to environmental changes, but recovered through yoga therapy practice.

2. Client Information

Physical Information: Female, Age 55 years, Height 162 cm, Weight 54 kg.

Occupation: Part-time sales staff.

Major Complaints: Pain in waist, shoulders, chest, and general stiffness in body.

Family Medical History: Father died from cerebral hemorrhage (age 49 years). Mother contracted diabetes mellitus (age 54 years) and died from gastrointestinal hemorrhage (age 84 years).

Diagnosis: She was diagnosed with rheumatoid arthritis at Hospital A in July of year X[41] (age 55 years).

Past Health Problems: Stomach ulcer (at age 22 years); Meniere's disease (at age 28 years); Intercostal neuralgia (at age 52 years).

History of Current Health Problems: This client suffered from poor health throughout much of her youth, but began yoga and became healthier. At fifty-one years of age, four years prior to starting yoga therapy, however, her husband had difficulty relating to people at work and retired early. He began spending a lot of time at home, and she felt she had to take care of him. She began feeling physical pain, and her body movements became robotic.

---

41 In all case studies in this book, "Year X" means the year the client began yoga therapy. Years prior to the start of yoga therapy are indicated with a minus, and years after the start of yoga therapy are indicated with a plus.

She sought treatment at a hospital and received injections. She also went for body work to relax her muscles and adjust her posture, but her symptoms did not change. At fifty-five years of age, she visited Hospital A and was diagnosed with rheumatoid arthritis. It was then that she also began yoga therapy.

Prescription Drugs: 100 mg Celecoxib, 2 capsules/day; 2 mg Methotrexate, 3 capsules/day; 5 mg Folic acid

Upbringing/Life Circumstances: She was raised in a small mountain village, and she lived with her grandparents, parents, and three siblings. She is the youngest of four. She left home at fifteen, married at twenty-two, and moved to Prefecture D. She worked as a dressmaker at home and raised two daughters. Her daughters have grown and left home, and she now lives with her husband.

Yoga Therapy History/Changes in Symptoms: She began yoga therapy once a week at a community center in Year X at fifty-five years of age. Each class was two hours. During her intake, she explained that she had rheumatoid arthritis in her legs and right arm, a swollen clavicle, and pain in the ribs. We obtained her informed consent to address her major complaints, then proceeded with initial tests. Her Ayurvedic Psychological Dosha Assessment (APDA) showed high rajas (95/150) and tamas (80/150). Her sattva score was low (40/150). Her General Health Questionnaire of Swami Vivekananda Yoga Anusandhana Samsthana (sVYASA) scores were 7/21 for physical health, 8/21 for emotional health, 8/21 for social health, and 5/21 for spiritual health, totaling 28/84 points (0–28 points is considered unhealthy; 29–55 healthy, 56–84 very healthy). Her POMS scores were tension/anxiety 58, depression 57, anger/hostility 56, fatigue 60, confusion 59. Her STAI scores were trait anxiety 47, state anxiety 52. On the SSIM-YSSMA (Yoga Sutra-Based State of Mind Assessment), she scored 5/5 for number 9 (instability of mind) (extremely unstable). We assessed that this was leading to disorders in the annamaya and vijnanamaya koshas. To assess misrecognition, we used the SSIM-YSAM (Yoga Sutra-based Assessment of Misrecognition), and she scored 5/5 for misrecognition of A (finite/infinite) and D (Self/non-Self).

The yoga therapist began instruction in breathing exercises without isometric resistance to avoid stressing her body. At the beginning of yoga therapy practice, the client felt pain and was unable to do the same movements as others in the class. After the client turned fifty-six, the yoga therapist added isometric resistance to the practice due to concern about the client's decreasing muscular strength. The client began practicing isometric asana to improve her range of motion, and she started yoga therapy counseling with regard to her relationship with her husband. By the following year, she was able to move smoothly and could do the same movements as others as her strength improved. After another year, she was able to carry heavier materials. Her cognition also changed. Her SSIM-YSAM score improved to 3/5 for both A (finite/infinite) and D (Self/non-Self). Her major symptoms of pain in her waist, shoulders, and chest and general stiffness decreased considerably.

As for medication, her doctor stopped prescribing Celecoxib (painkiller) when she was fifty-six years old. Her CRP level (inflammation indicator) changed from 3.81 mg (age 55 years) to 0.29 mg after two years of yoga therapy (less than 0.2 mg is considered normal). In year $X + 3$ (age 58 years), all pain in her waist, shoulders, and chest disappeared, although some stiffness remained. Her POMS tension/anxiety decreased from 58 to 39, depression 57 to 49, anger/hostility 56 to 39, and confusion 59 to 49. Her STAI trait anxiety decreased from 47 to 40, and state anxiety 52 to 35, indicting normal conditions. On the sVYASA General Health Questionnaire, her scores improved as follows: physical health from 7 to 15 of 21, emotional health from 8 to 15/21, social health from 8 to 11/21, spiritual health from 5 to 18/21, totaling 58/84 to put her in the "very healthy" bracket. Her SSIM-YSSMA scores decreased from 5/5 for instability of mind to 2/5. SSIM-YSAM (misrecognition of finite for infinite, non-self for Self) both decreased to 2/5. Her APDA rajas score improved to 70/150, tamas to 60/150, and sattva 100/150.

Client Testimony: I could not accept my diagnosis for rheumatoid arthritis because I had finally become healthy practicing yoga. Then while living with my retired husband, I lost confidence. After practicing yoga therapy, I learned to accept my illness and then started recovering. I tried to keep all my difficulties to myself, but gradually I started asking others for help. From now on, I want to manage my rheumatoid arthritis by exercising self-control.

3. Observations

The pain from rheumatoid arthritis led the client to change from being positive to negative. After starting yoga therapy, her physical strength increased as did her body weight. She became able to see things more objectively and change the way she thought about herself and her husband. She saw her rheumatoid arthritis in a different light and gained mental strength. The yoga therapist used both conventional psychological tests and YTA tools, and then applied yoga therapy techniques to address the client's cognition in the vijnanamaya kosha, and visible changes were seen in her physical symptoms.

FICTIONAL CASE STUDY 2: YOGA THERAPY FOR HYPOTHYROIDISM

1. Introduction

Hypothyroidism (Hashimoto's thyroiditis) is a condition in which the thyroid gland does not produce enough of certain important hormones. Body processes slow down with insufficient thyroid hormone, making metabolism sluggish. Symptoms of Hashimoto's thyroiditis include weakness, weight gain, sensitivity to cold, cold hands and feet, fatigue, dry skin, brittle nails, and thinning, brittle hair. Other early symptoms include muscle achiness, joint pain, and heavy menstrual periods. Women, especially those older than sixty years, are more likely to have hypothyroidism. This client suffered from Hashimoto's thyroiditis and reported improvement in her symptoms after six months of yoga therapy practice.

2. **Client Information**

Physical information: Female, Age 61 years, Height 155 cm, Weight 58 kg.

Occupation: Part-time college instructor.

Major Complaints: Daytime sleepiness, insomnia, weight gain, sensitivity to cold, cold hands and feet, fatigue, dizziness.

Family Medical History: Parent (age 89 years) high blood pressure.

Past Health Problems: None.

Diagnosis: Year X – 10 January (age 51 years) Hashimoto's thyroiditis Hospital A.

History of Current Health Problems: In January year X – 10 (age 51 years), she felt discomfort in the throat, fatigue, and weight gain. She visited Hospital A and was diagnosed with Hashimoto's thyroiditis and began taking medication. In December year X – 1 (age 60 years) she started having difficulty going out because of daytime sleepiness and fatigue. She slept badly and woke up several times at night. She also felt cold even if she put on warm clothes. In April year X (age 61 years), she started practicing yoga therapy.

Upbringing/Life Circumstances: Raised in a healthy family in the United States. After graduating from college she got a job at a university. She married in year X – 33 (age 28 years) and moved to Japan following her husband's job transfer in year X – 8 (age 53 years). She felt severe stress from life in a foreign country and also worried about her elderly parent and son in the United States. In year X – 4 (age 57 years), her son had a sudden illness, and she made several return trips between Japan and the United States.

Yoga Therapy History/Changes in Symptoms: She began yoga therapy ninety minutes once a week at a community center in April year X (age 61 years). During her first intake she spoke of severe stress due to phone calls every day from her mother and her concern for her son's health. She also explained that she snacked between meals. We obtained her informed consent to address her complaints, and first used the SSIM-YSSMA (Yoga Sutra-based State of Mind Assessment). She scored 5/5 in number 8 (inability) and number 9 (instability of mind). To assess misrecognition, we used the SSIM-YSAM (Yoga Sutra-based Assessment of Misrecognition). She scored 4/5 in D (Self/non-Self misrecognition), which came from the conflict in her parent-child relationship. She was losing sight of herself due to difficulty fulfilling the responsibilities of daughter-wife-mother roles. On the sVYASA General Health Questionnaire, she scored 15/21 for A (physical health), 12/21 for B (emotional health), 12/21 for C (social health), 15/21 for D (spiritual health), to total 54/84 points. Her POMS showed tension 70, depression 50, anger 45, vigor 40, fatigue 65, confusion 50. And the Ayurveda Dosha Test (prakrti) showed (V) vata 28 points, (P) pitta 20 points, (K) kapha 38 points, 38/86 = 0.44 (kapha predominant). The dosha balance (vikrti) test showed (V) vata 35 points, (P) pitta 11 points, (K) kapha 28 points, vata predominant. The APDA (for clients' use) showed rajas mark 26/150 and tamas mark 12/150.

We started her with isometric breathing exercises, isometric sukshma vyayama, cyclic meditation techniques and some pranayama. We also used isometric asana and vedic meditation (shravana, manana, nididhyasana, and jnana). We did ninety-minutes of yoga counseling with Shinkan meditation once a month. After five months in September Year X, the client started to feel bodily relaxation and reduction in other complaints, especially dizziness. At this time the changes in data were as follows: sVYA-SA General Health Questionnaire A 16(+1), B 15(+3), C 15(+3), D 18(+2), total 64 (+9). POMS: tension 41 (–29), depression 45 (–5), anger 40 (–5), vigor 45 (+5), fatigue 49 (–16), confusion 38 (–12). Dosha balance (vikrti) test showed that (V) vata 30 points, (P) pitta 20 points, (K) kapha 36 points. Vata decreased, and kapha increased. And the APDA (for clients' use) showed rajas mark 20(–6)/150 and tamas mark 10(-2)/150.

Her SSIM-YSSMA scores changed to the most healthy marks in number 8 (inability) and number 9 (instability of mind) to 1/5 points. Also the SSIM-YSAM D (Self/non-Self misrecognition) marks decreased to 1/5 points. The client could breathe deeply and felt improvement in cold sensitivity, cold hands and feet. The day-time yoga therapy practice and isometric exercises relieved insomnia and her fatigue was resolved.

Client Testimony: I can feel my body move comfortably. If I move during the day, I can sleep well at night. While I practice yoga therapy, I feel my body warm and forget about dizziness and sensitivity to cold. I feel my mind calm down after Veda and Shinkan meditation. My health condition has improved, and I can enjoy walking and yoga exercise. I also enjoy daily pranayama practice. My fatigue improved and my muscle mass increased, so I think my metabolism is improving too. I did not know I was so full of anxiety and discontent, but after meditation, I feel much calmer. I had homework after each yoga therapy session, and I really enjoyed it. My anxiety dramatically reduced and my relationship with my mother is much better now.

3. Observations

This client had difficulty concentrating in her yoga therapy practice at the beginning because of her dizziness. But after she mastered deep breathing she could relax and could concentrate better. One of the reasons her symptoms improved is that she appreciated and had a positive attitude toward her practice.

CHAPTER 2

Yoga Therapy Assessment (YTA) and Yoga Therapy

Instruction (YTI) for the Pranamaya Kosha

1) Yoga Therapy's Pathogenesis Theory and the Pranamaya Kosha

THE BREATH IS OFTEN SPOKEN of as the bridge between body and mind. The pranamaya kosha can also be considered a bridge between the three inner koshas and the food sheath (physical body). As explained in the previous section, in yoga, the source of disease is in the buddhi, one of the four psychological organs (the driver of the chariot), and it is responsible for recognition, discrimination, prediction, decision, and executive instruction. After receiving information, the buddhi guides the manas (the reins of the human chariot) to steer the organs of perception and action (the ten horses). Any problem with information sent from the buddhi to the manas will affect the movement of the reins and the ten horses. As a result, the hypothalamus, which regulates breathing, will also be affected, as will be the functioning of the autonomic nervous system, endocrine and immune systems. This can then lead to problems in cardiovascular functions and breathing irregularities. In this way, the pranamaya kosha is affected by the malfunction of the buddhi and manas, and disrupted breathing can in turn lead to physical manifestations of disease.

Yoga therapists assess clients based on this understanding of the relationship among the koshas. This has already been explained in the section on the annamaya kosha. If it is possible to remove the cause of disruption,

Yoga Therapy Theory

then yoga therapy has the potential to eliminate the fundamental cause of disease. Much about a client's condition can be learned from observing the breath.

2) YOGA THERAPY ASSESSMENT (YTA) OF THE PRANAMAYA KOSHA

Here, I will introduce some of the assessment methods for the pranamaya kosha to confirm whether the nine causes of distraction in the mind that Patanjali lists as obstacles—disease, languor, doubt, carelessness, laziness, worldly-mindedness, delusion, nonachievement of a stage, and instability—are affecting the pranamaya kosha. You can also try practicing these assessment methods yourself.

A. CHECKING RESPIRATORY FUNCTION (ALEXISOMIA)

* Once a month, yoga therapists should measure the maximum length of the client's exhalation. This can be done by timing how long the client can continue to say, "ooo," and check to see if the length of exhalation continues to increases with yoga therapy practice or not.
* Yoga therapists can check to see whether the client is able to be aware of movement in the abdomen, chest and shoulders while doing sectional breathing.

B. SELF-ASSESSMENT TO CHECK AWARENESS OF NATURAL BREATH

* Place one finger under your nose and try to feel the flow of the breath in and out of the nostrils.
* Place your palm in front of your half-opened mouth. Feel the flow of the natural breath.
* Be aware of the natural flow of the breath on the upper lip or at the tip of the nose.

3) Principles of Yoga Therapy Instruction (YTI) for the Pranamaya Kosha

Yoga therapy for the pranamaya kosha involves voluntary control of breathing and is, therefore, fundamental training in self-awareness. Controlling the breath influences the central nervous system, and thus relates to control of the endocrine and immune systems. In this way, yoga therapy techniques for the pranamaya kosha have a larger and more direct impact on subtler physiological functions than practices for the physical body, the annamaya kosha.

To practice pranayama safely, it is important to first decide which technique to use, and identify the strength, speed, and the number of repetitions that are suitable for your current condition. You could start with the exercises and number of repetitions introduced in the chapter on the annamaya kosha at the end of the anti-ageing or isometric yoga therapy programs. It is best, however, if you can first be instructed by a qualified yoga therapist.

Now, I will introduce some of the teachings in the scriptures relating to pranayama. You will get a sense for the depth of this traditional wisdom that has been handed down over thousands of years.

―――

REFERENCE 4: GUIDANCE FROM THE SCRIPTURES
Mahatma Svatmarama's *Hatha Yoga Pradipika*

Chapter 2 Pranayama, Verse 15

Just as a lion, an elephant, or a tiger is tamed by degrees, similarly respiration is to be brought under control gradually; otherwise, it would harm the aspirant.

Commentary: Traditionally, the guru would decide the number of repetitions, intensity, and speed of pranayama techniques. In the case of yoga therapy, therapists must select the technique and the suitable number of repetitions, intensity, and speed of pranayama practices based on the assessment of the client's body and mind. Even in traditional yoga, learning to control the breath is a gradual practice. In my case as well, my guru was very careful in instructing us to practice for three to six months before increasing the length of the breath, even by one second. Because yoga therapists are generally teaching people with health issues, therapists must be very careful in monitoring how clients respond to pranayama exercise. It is a dangerous mistake to assume that increasing the number of repetitions for a pranayama practice that shows good results will make the client even healthier. Please be aware that many adverse events happen in relation to the pranamaya kosha. For actual pranayama practice, please receive instruction from a qualified therapist.

Chapter 2 Verse 16

By proper practice of pranayama, all diseases are annihilated. Improper practice of pranayama (on the other hand) gives rise to all sorts of diseases.

Commentary: As stated in this verse, "all diseases are annihilated" when traditional yoga is practiced correctly, as it harmonizes our endocrine, immune, and nervous systems, creating what we call the "triangle of homeostasis." It is believed that the ancient yogis were aware of this from their own experience. For this reason, pranayama is introduced in yoga therapy practices, but only after the therapist has assessed the client's mental and physical condition and designed a suitable practice. As the client's capacity changes over time, the number of repetitions, intensity, and speed of pranayama are also adjusted accordingly.

From ancient times, yogis first acquired a certain level of mastery in asana, and then went on to master their indriyas (organs of perception and action), exercising moderation in their diet, and following their guru's instructions in pranayama. In yoga therapy as well, it is necessary to adjust the practice to the ability of the client. *Hatha Yoga Pradipika* chapter 2 verse 2 says, "When prana moves, chitta (the mental force) moves. When prana is without movement, chitta is without movement. By this (steadiness of prana) the yogi attains steadiness and should thus restrain the vayu (air)."

It is thus evident that the ancient yogis knew that the function of breathing is the bridge between the physical body and functions of the mind. For this reason, pranayama plays a central role in the mind-body practices of yoga therapy, and therapists are very careful in their instruction. If practiced skillfully, pranayama practice can help keep balance and harmony between body and mind to maintain good health.

4) Prevention of Adverse Events in the Pranamaya Kosha

Pranayama is a very effective method to induce physiological changes in the body and to influence the mind, and for that very reason, careless practice must be avoided. I will list some points of caution that yoga therapists should consider in order to prevent adverse events. If you are interested in practicing yourself, consult with a qualified yoga therapist to select the best practice for your condition.

1. Pranayama programs must be made in accordance with the physical ability and motivation of the practitioner.
2. Pranayama should be instructed in a way that enables clients to practice safely at home by themselves. Yoga therapists should ensure that clients do not stray from the prescribed number of practice sessions and repetitions.

Yoga Therapy Theory

③ Pranayama should be done before meals or one to two hours after meals. Yoga therapists must caution clients against practicing immediately after meals.

④ Posture is important in breathing exercises, and the spine should be lengthened. It is appropriate to sit on a cushion to raise the buttocks off the floor, or to sit in a chair.

⑤ If any adverse events occur as a result of the practice, stop the practice for a few days and if necessary, consult a more experienced yoga therapist.

⑥ Do not exert undue force or strain during the practice. Clients should be aware of their own life force and energy when practicing yoga therapy.

⑦ Every few months, check for changes in vital data, such as the length of the client's exhalation (by measuring the length of exhaling with the sound "nnn"). Monitor physical changes so that practices can be adjusted in a way most suitable for the client.

⑧ Kumbhaka (holding the breath) is not included in yoga therapy instruction. Do not instruct clients in kumbhaka.

5) Physiological Changes and Pranayama

Pranayama induces many physiological changes in our bodies and has a strong influence on the mind. I will include summaries of some research that investigated the physiological impacts of pranayama. Yoga therapists need to know what physical and physiological changes can be expected from each practice. I would encourage you to read the research papers introduced here and practice pranayama after having understood the effects written in them.

A. Decrease in Serum Cortisol during Yoga Exercise Is Correlated with Alpha-Wave Activation[42]

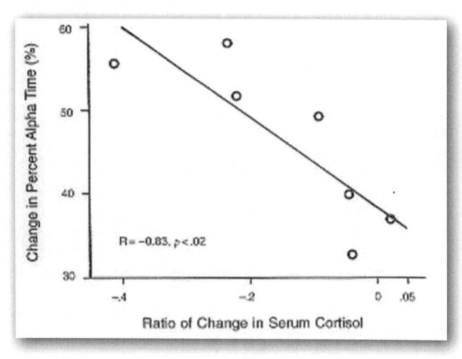

The Japan Yoga Therapy Society conducted basic medical research that showed that regular practice of yoga therapy is effective for the management of stress and hypertension. This graph shows that the more alpha time for practitioners who did sixty minutes of Hatha Yoga, the greater the reduction in adrenocortical hormone (cortisol), which indicates a reduction in stress. When clients experienced a stressful condition, the adrenocortical hormone was secreted from the pituitary gland. This figure shows that when concentration was good and the relative frequency of alpha waves was high, secretion of adrenocorticotrophic hormone (ACTH) decreased and clients were able to stay in a mind-body condition that was more relaxed than usual. Moreover, blood pressure was reduced when

---

42 Tsutomu Kamei et al., "Decrease in Serum Cortisol during Yoga Exercise Is Correlated with Alpha Wave Activation," *Perceptual and Motor Skills* 90, no. 3 (2000): 1027–32.

Yoga Therapy Theory

there was a decrease in the secretion of ACTH, a hormone that increases blood pressure.

B. Correlation between Appearance Ratio of Alpha Waves and Yoga Therapy[43]

The diagram that follows shows the appearance ratio of alpha waves after practicing a Hatha Yoga program. The program included ten minutes of rest with the eyes closed, ten minutes of Hatha Yoga exercises, fifteen minutes of pranayama, and twenty minutes of So-Ham meditation. We examined the alpha-wave appearance ratio in the four stages of the program. Seven cases out of eight showed increased alpha waves during Hatha Yoga, but all cases showed increased alpha-wave appearance in pranayama. During the twenty minutes of So-Ham meditation, some showed increased and some showed decreased alpha waves depending on the level of skill. This paper, "The Activation of Cellular Immunity by Correlation between Pranayama and the Changes of Alpha Waves in the Brain" received an award at the seventh Japan Holistic Medical Society Conference in November 2006.

---

43 Tsutomu Kamei, Kohji Murata, Nobutaka Suzuki, and Keishin Kimura, "The Meaning of Yoga 'Recombination': A Discussion of Immunological Change in Yogic Practice" (International Conference on Mind Body Science: Physical and Physiological Approach joint with the Eighteenth Symposium on Life Information Science), *Journal of International Society of Life Information Science* 22, no. 2 (2004): 392–98.

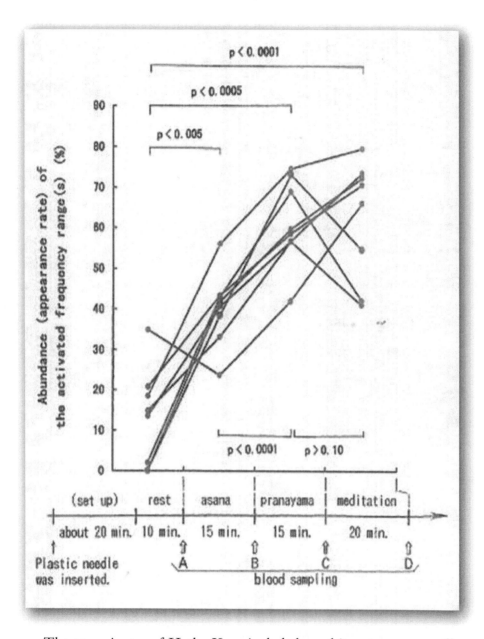

The ten minutes of Hatha Yoga included paschimottanasana, ardha matsyendrasana, bhujangasana, matsyasana, and dhanurasana. Shavasana was done after each pose.

Fifteen minutes of pranayama was practiced as follows (with thirty seconds of rest between each exercise):

1. Thirty seconds of sukha pranayama: slow inhalation and exhalation through both nostrils
2. Thirty seconds of agni prasarana (one breath per second), followed by thirty seconds of rest
3. Ninety seconds of surya vedana: inhalation through the right nostril and exhalation through the left nostril
4. Ninety seconds of chandra vedana: inhalation through the left nostril and exhalation through the right nostril
5. Two minutes of nadi shuddhi: alternate nostril breathing
6. Three minutes of ujjayi pranayama: breathing through both nostrils with awareness of the sound of friction in the throat
7. Bhramari for 2.5 minutes: both nostrils

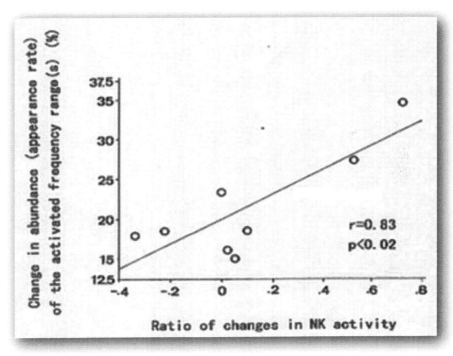

C. Correlation of Yogic Breathing Exercise and the Activation of Natural Killer (NK) Cells[44]

In this research, various changes were examined after fifteen minutes of pranayama. Examination of the results showed a positive correlation between increased NK-cell activity and alpha-wave appearance. There was also an inverse correlation in secretion of adrenocortical hormone (a stress hormone) and alpha-wave appearance. It is possible that this inverse correlation is the reason for NK-cell activity, but because it happened in a short fifteen minutes, we speculate that NK-cell activity was more likely stimulated by the opioids released in the brain during pranayama. Whatever the reason, we were encouraged to see an increase in NK-cell activity with fifteen minutes of pranayama, and will continue research to investigate the significance of these findings.

D. Correlation between Yogic Breathing Exercise and Antioxidant Ability[45]

In our research with people exposed to radiation from the Chernobyl nuclear accident, we found that six months of isometric yoga breathing exercises for twenty minutes a day increased antioxidant ability and decreased oxidant stress levels.

---

44 Tsutomu Kamei, Kohji Murata, Nobutaka Suzuki, and Keishin Kimura, "Correlation between Alpha Rhythms and Natural Killer Cell Activity during Yogic Respiratory Exercise," *Stress and Health* 17 (2001): 141–45, doi; 10.1002/smi.889.

45 Tsutomu Kamei et al., *The Isometric Yogic Breathing Exercise Routine for Half a Year Increases Anti-Oxidant Ability.* Paper presented at the 12th International Congress of Behavior Medicine, Budapest, Hungary. Aug 2012.

Yoga Therapy Theory

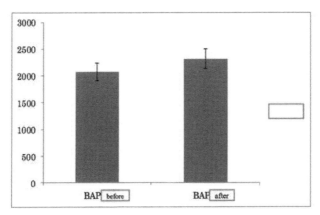

(The Changes of Anti-oxidant ability: BAP test)
[μ Mol / l] by Isometric Yogic Breathing Exercise for 6 month (n=17)

Kamei T.et. al. 12th International Congress of Behavioral Medicine

Chart 1. Isometric yogic breathing exercise for six months, twenty minutes per day, increased the antioxidant ability of people exposed to radiation from the Chernobyl nuclear accident, and their oxidant-stress levels decreased. From this, we infer that isometric yogic breathing exercise may be useful in slowing down the ageing process.

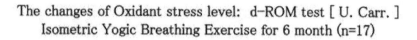

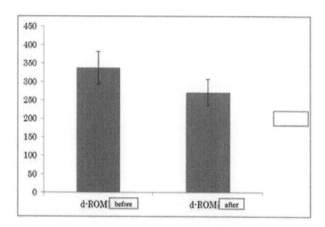

(Kamei T. et. al. 12th International Congress of Behavioral Medicine)

Chart 2. The results indicate that the yogic breathing exercises increased the secretion of a neurotransmitter into the blood, increasing cellular immunity. This change in the blood shows similarities to the effects seen in the first study introduced on changes in serum cortisol and alpha-time percentage. After six months of practicing yoga therapy, the amount of active oxygen in the blood decreased from abnormally high to normal levels. We presented this research at the twelfth International Congress of Behavioral Medicine in Budapest in August 2012.

6) Fictional Case Studies: Pranamaya Kosha

Information from several real case studies was compiled into the fictional cases that follow in order to illustrate some of the results we have seen in stress reduction after practicing yoga therapy. In these case reports, several Semi-Structured Interview Manual (SSIM) results are introduced. The reason for including them is not only to show how yoga therapy practice can improve people's conditions, but we at JYTS are very pleased with the promise the SSIMs are showing as both assessment and monitoring tools. They may be one way to ground yoga therapy in the thousands of years of yogic wisdom that tends to be overlooked in comparison to conventional medicine and clinical psychology.

FICTIONAL CASE STUDY 3: YOGA THERAPY FOR BRONCHIAL ASTHMA

1. **Introduction**

Bronchial asthma is an illness with paroxysmal attacks of breathing difficulties with repeated wheezing and coughing. The cause of this asthma is inflammation and hypersensitivity in the respiratory tract. Attacks are attributed to inhalation of antigens, over exercise, infection, and stress. This is a case study of a man who suffered bronchial asthma for many years and who got pneumonia. After doing yoga therapy, he became more aware of his own condition and was freed from previous stresses.

2. **Client Information**

Physical Information: Male, Age 51 years, Height 175 cm, Weight 67 kg.

Occupation: Certified level-1 architect.

Major Complaints: Asthma attacks, respiratory distress, back pain, cold hands and feet.

Family Medical History: Father (age 85 years) gout, high blood pressure, cataract; mother (age 80 years) leg catheterization, osteoarthritis in the knee (artificial joint replacement), and glaucoma.

Diagnosis: Year X - 21 (age 30 years) bronchial asthma Hospital A.

Past Health Problems: Sinusitis (age 13 years), Herpes zoster, gout (age 44 years), *Staphylococcus aureus* pneumonia (age 50 years).

History of Current Health Problems: In year X - 21 (age 30 years), he worked very long hours, sometimes through the night. He developed symptoms of coughing and breathing difficulties. He was diagnosed with bronchial asthma at Hospital A, and referred to National Health Center B, where he had blood tests done every two months. In year X - 7 (age 44 years) he was transferred to another section of his company and developed herpes zoster and gout. In May of year X - 1 (age 50 years), he had many business trips and worked long overtime hours. His cough did not stop, and he was diagnosed with *S. aureus* at Medical Center C and hospitalized for a month. Then he had home treatment for a while before returning to work. In year X (age 51 years) his friend introduced him to yoga therapy. In year X + 1 (age 52 years), he developed cataracts.

Upbringing/Life Circumstances: He is the youngest of three brothers. His father owned a construction materials company that had been handed down over several generations. His mother was very strict regarding his education. After graduating from college, he worked at an interior design company. He worked in its construction section because he was licensed as an architect, but his section was closed when the company changed its business practices. Because of restructuring and reduced personnel, he was assigned to many business trips and had to work long overtime hours. In May of year X - 1 (age 50 years), he developed a constant cough. His personality was such that he could not refuse when asked to do something, so he accepted all work assignments even when he was already overextended. In October of year X - 1 (age 50 years), he was diagnosed with *S. aureus* and hospitalized for one month. After that he had home treatment, then returned to work. He lives with his wife (age 46 years) and one daughter (age 10 years).

Yoga Therapy History/Changes in Symptoms: He started ed practicing yoga therapy in November year X (age 51 years).

During the intake, he listed his symptoms as asthmatic attacks, respiratory distress, back pain, and cold hands and feet. He also talked about overwork. He gave informed consent to practice yoga therapy to address his complaints, and we began initial tests. His APDA showed his sattva was 50/150, rajas 80/150, and tamas 120/150. His SOC (Sense of Coherence) mental test score was a low 120/203, so we assessed that he had a tamas predominant mind, and his tolerance for stress was quite low. Considering the results of initial tests, we used the SSIM-BGAK (Bhagavad Gita-based Assessment of Karma). He scored a low 2/5 for "ability to see beyond polarity," and we assessed that his vijnanamaya kosha was unbalanced. We began his yoga therapy with chair breathing exercises and also asked him to practice at home. During the first assessment, his complexion was unhealthy and his hands and feet cold. He had difficulty with pranayama and breathed through his mouth. In accordance with the assessment, we instructed him in cyclic meditation. In February year X + 1 (age 52 years), he said his throat had less phlegm, and his hands and feet were warmer. His back pain improved. His yoga therapy practice was adjusted to include OM meditation and isometric asana and other pranayama. In accordance with the changes in his condition, in March of year X + 1 (age 52 years), his medication was reduced to pre-hospitalization levels. In April year X + 1 (age 52 years), his asthma attacks stopped and he breathed more easily. The same year, his blood sugar level rose because of medication, and he developed cataracts, but after changing dosage, his blood-sugar level returned to normal. Currently (December year X + 1, age 52 years) he is taking montelukast/clarithromycin/salmeterol and xinafoate/fluticasone propionate for asthma, and benzbromarone for gout. He became more aware of his own condition and started saying he should not work too hard. His new SSIM-BGAK score for "ability to see beyond polarity" increased to 4/5, and his APDA score for sattva improved to 100/150, rajas 70/150, and tamas 70/150. We assessed that there was improvement in the balance of his five koshas.

Client Testimony: I don't get much exercise, so I feel refreshed when I practice yoga. During yoga and after I finish, it is easier to clear my throat of phlegm. I have felt more relaxed since I have time to check in with myself. I felt tension when I worked in the office, but I decided to relax more at work. I want to continue practicing yoga.

3. Observations

This practitioner did not exercise much and had little awareness of his own mind-body condition. He was very serious and a perfectionist at work. He often looked negative during initial yoga therapy. Over time, he started seeing things in a more positive light. Yoga therapy facilitates better mind-body awareness, and therefore facilitates improved health. The above-mentioned clinical psychology tests indicated the same improvements. His blood pressure increased after yoga therapy, and we see this as an improvement in his autonomic nervous system functions (from primarily parasympathetic to more sympathetic). Increased ease in clearing his throat also indicates more predominance of his sympathetic nervous system. He is still taking various kinds of medicine, but his mentality and recognition normalized, so we can expect continued improvement.

Fictional Case Study 4: Yoga Therapy for Chronic Obstructive Pulmonary Disease (COPD)

1. Introduction

Cigarette smoking is the leading cause of COPD. Most people who have COPD smoke or used to smoke. Long-term exposure to other lung irritants—such as air pollution, chemical fumes, or dust—also may contribute to COPD. Symptoms of COPD often worsen over time and can limit ability to do routine activities. Severe COPD may prevent even basic activities like walking, cooking, or taking care of oneself. Most of the time, COPD is diagnosed in middle-aged or older adults. COPD has no cure, and doctors do not know how to reverse the damage to the airways and lungs. However, treatments and lifestyle changes can help one feel better, stay more active, and slow the progress of the disease. This practitioner was diagnosed with COPD and was advised not to smoke by his doctor, but he could not stop. The yoga therapist suggested he do yoga therapy pranayama. After five months practice his lung capacity recovered.

2. **Client Information**

Physical Information: Male, Age 65 years, Height 168 cm, Weight 68kg.

Occupation: Pensioner.

Major Complaints: Shortness of breath, insomnia, fatigue, habitual smoking.

Family Medical History: Father died in traffic accident (age 40 years); mother died at childbirth (age 35 years).

Diagnosis: February year X (age 65 years) COPD Hospital A, Doctor B.

Past Health Problems: Stomach ulcer (age 30 years); Meniere's disease (age 61 years).

History of Current Health Problems: In year X - 3 (age 62 years), he started to feel fatigue and could not do long hours of work. He was smoking thirty-six cigarettes a day, and was told to quit. He was worried about his dark complexion after being told he looked ten years older than his actual age. He tried to quit smoking but failed. His wife was then diagnosed with lung disease due to passive smoking. In April year X (age 65 years), his friend, a yoga therapist, advised him to practice breathing exercises. He tried and felt some improvement in his health condition, so he decided to practice yoga therapy in earnest.

Upbringing/Life Circumstances: He lost his parents when he was young, and his aunt raised him and his younger sister. At nineteen years of age, he found a job in a shipyard and left home. At thirty-one years of age, he married a coworker. They had two children. He had been smoking for forty-six years since the age of nineteen. After he had an accident badly hitting his head at his work place, he returned to his hometown and started to work in construction. He retired in year X - 10 (age 55 years). Presently, he lives with his wife, mother-in-law, and two daughters.

Yoga Therapy History/Changes in Symptoms: From February to July of year X (age 65 years), he practiced yoga therapy at his home for twenty to sixty minutes. During the first intake, he mentioned his major complaints, and gave us his informed consent to use yoga therapy to address the complaints. His STAI showed high state anxiety at 41 points, and normal trait anxiety at 33 points. His systolic blood pressure was 122 mmHg and diastolic pressure 95 mmHg. His heart rate was 63/minute, and respiration was 14 bpm (breaths per minute). Considering the information from his initial tests, we used the SSIM-AS (Assessment of Spirituality). Results were 1/5 for A (ability to regulate attachment/obsessiveness). We assessed that mental weakness was one reason for his excessive smoking. We started his yoga therapy program with yoga therapy pranayama, using breathing exercises and sukshma vyayama with sound in the sitting or supine position to help him become aware of his attachments. Each practice was about twenty minutes. After two months, he had reduced pain in his right shoulder. Average bio-data showed systolic pressure changed from 122 to 136 mmHg (+14) and diastolic pressure from 95 to 90 mmHg (-5). Heart rate decreased from 63 to 59 (-4) times per minute. He said his breathing felt smoother. He began voluntarily practicing yoga therapy every day for fifteen minutes. After this, during counseling, it became clear he had anxiety about ageing. We added isometric asana breathing for anti-ageing effects. In June year X, he began increasing physical activity. He felt some difficulty breathing while working, but began recovering more quickly. He began volunteering for traffic safety. During his final psychological assessment in July year X, his state anxiety changed from 41 to 26, and trait anxiety from 33 to 29, and his major complaints of shortness of breath, insomnia, and fatigue improved. His smoking had also greatly reduced. In August year X he did not smoke, so we conducted an SSIM-AS assessment, and his ability to regulate attachment/obsessiveness showed strong ability at 4/5. His family members praised him, and his relationship with them improved.

Client Testimony: When is I was sixty-two years old, people told me I looked seventy because of the way I breathed, my complexion, and how easily I got fatigued. I was shocked. Then I was diagnosed with COPD after getting a lung CT scan, and the doctor told me not to smoke. I also had insomnia. I bought a product at the drugstore to help me stop smoking, but it did not work. Then someone recommended yoga therapy. After I started it, I felt refreshed in my brain, as if smog was clearing up. So I started yoga therapy practice seriously, and I did not want to smoke anymore. This feeling was so strange to me. My complexion improved and my family is happy, and I am really grateful to my yoga therapy practice.

3. **Observations**

This practitioner initially did not take care of his body or health, and was not aware of his shortness of breath. Smoking increased risk factors. After starting yoga therapy, especially yogic breathing exercises, he gradually was able to exhale deeply, which he had not been able to do before. His complexion improved. This indicates that the yoga therapy practice promoted his lung capacity, which eased his breathing difficulties as a COPD patient. In addition, his self-control improved and he successfully stopped smoking. He was able to cultivate his mind and became aware of his mind-body connection. These changes improved his state and trait anxiety. He became more cheerful and more at peace. His quality of life improved.

CHAPTER 3

Yoga Therapy Assessment (YTA) and Yoga Therapy Instruction (YTI) for the Manomaya Kosha

1) Yoga Therapy's Pathogenesis Theory and the Manomaya Kosha

THE MANOMAYA KOSHA IS COMPRISED of the manas (mind) and the ten indriyas. The indriyas are often referred to as "sense organs," but may be better understood as the five abilities to perceive (abilities to see, hear, touch, taste, and smell), and the five abilities to take action (grasping, locomotion, reproduction, excretion, and speech). Disturbances and illness in the pranamaya and annamaya koshas arise when the ability of the ten indriyas to collect information and communicate with the buddhi, the discriminating intellect of the vijnanamaya kosha, is compromised.

Explaining in terms of the human chariot theory, when the driver (buddhi/vijnanamaya kosha) does not skillfully hold the reins (manas/manomaya kosha) to control the ten horses (indriyas/manomaya kosha), the horses get out of control, and disease may result as it causes disruptions in the entire system. *Katha Upanishad* Verse 1.3.5 explains this state of mind as, "When a person lacks discrimination and his mind is undisciplined, the senses run hither and thither like wild horses."

The image of ten wild horses creating havoc for a chariot driver struggling to control the reins, thus disrupting the whole body of the chariot and disturbing any occupants is a metaphor that makes it quite easy to understand the role of the manomaya kosha in the development of disease.

Following is an explanation of how to assess the manomaya kosha. It is a very specialized assessment.

2) Yoga Therapy Assessment (YTA) and the Manomaya Kosha

After asking the client for medical history and symptoms and assessing any functional problems in the physical body, it is necessary to assess the client's ten indriyas, the five abilities to perceive (jnana indriya) and five abilities to take action (karma indriya). This is done by assessing the client's sensory and motor capacity, using the *Semi-Structured Interview Manual—Assessment of the Indriyas* (SSIM-AI). The SSIM-AI contains questions that the yoga therapist can ask the client regarding each jnana and karma indriya and score how well or poorly each indriya is functioning. Tabulating the scores gives an overall assessment of the manomaya kosha. Yoga therapists certified by JYTS are educated in how to use this SSIM-AI.

Though yoga therapists may not have the same specialized education as physical therapists, assessment of physical functions related to the ten indriyas is necessary within the range of common sense in order to provide effective and safe yoga therapy. I will explain part of this assessment below.

1. *Organs of perception*: assess faculties of taste, sight, hearing, touch, smell
2. *Organs of action*: assess functions of hands, feet, reproductive organs, excretory organs, speech organs
   * Clients are instructed in simple asana and pranayama exercises to assess their awareness of strength, flexibility and position of arms and legs.
   * Clients are asked questions to assess their objective awareness of reproductive and excretory functions.

* Clients are asked questions to assess their awareness of what they intend to say.

As I explained earlier, the *Katha Upanishad* describes the human system as a chariot drawn by ten horses, what I refer to as the human chariot theory. In this Upanishad, there are verses we use for assessing the condition of manomaya kosha. Some have already been mentioned in a previous chapter, but I will review them again.

REFERENCE 5: *KATHA UPANISHAD* PART 1 CHAPTER 3

Verse 3: *Know the Self as lord of the chariot, the body as the chariot itself, the discriminating intellect as the charioteer, and the mind as reins.*

Verse 4:*The senses, say the wise, are the horses; selfish desires are the roads they travel. When the Self is confused with the body, mind, and senses, they point out, he seems to enjoy pleasure and suffer sorrow.*

Verse 5:*When a person lacks discrimination and his mind is undisciplined, the senses run hither and thither like wild horses.*

Verse 6: *But they obey the rein like trained horses when one has discrimination and has made the mind one-pointed.*

Verse 7: *Those who lack discrimination, with little control over their thoughts and far from pure, reach not the pure state of immortality but wander from death to death*

Verse 8: *But those who have discrimination, with a still mind and a pure heart, reach journey's end, never again to fall into the jaws of death.*

Verse 9: *With a discriminating intellect as charioteer and a trained mind as reins, they attain the supreme goal of life, to be united with the Lord of Love.*

Verse 10: *The senses derive from objects of sense perception, sense objects from mind, mind from intellect, and intellect from ego;*

Verse 11: *Ego from undifferentiated consciousness, and consciousness from Brahman. Brahman is the First Cause and last refuge.*

Verse 12: *Brahman, the hidden Self in everyone, does not shine forth. He is revealed only to those who keep their minds one-pointed on the Lord of Love and thus develop a superconscious manner of knowing.*

Commentary: From a historical point of view, the *Katha Upanishad* was written one to two thousand years before the *Yoga Sutras*. It is clear that the methods of controlling the mind and body described in the *Yoga Sutras* have their origin in older scriptures, such as this *Katha Upanishad*. A more detailed explanation of the *Katha Upanishad* is in part I chapter II section 2 in this book.

Even thousands of years ago, the importance of the intellect's control over sense organs was understood, and in our modern society, this wisdom is of immense importance in addressing the many unhealthy ways in which we try to handle stress. I believe yoga therapists are making a valuable contribution to society by teaching stress management based on these ancient teachings.

––––––

3) Principles of Yoga Therapy Instruction (YTI) and the Manomaya Kosha

The ability of the buddhi to perceive objectively the activities of the ten sense organs makes up the foundation of YTI theory for the manomaya kosha. The manas (mind/reins) and ten indriya (organs of perception and action) have a tendency to look outward. Turning their attention inward is the goal of yoga therapy for the manomaya kosha.

Yoga therapy techniques for the manomaya kosha include various breathing exercises (pranayama), controlling the senses (pratyahara), and methods of concentration (dharana). Meditation techniques from Raja Yoga and Vedic meditation can also be used. They enable the client to gain self-control, both physically and mentally, through counseling, psychoeducation, and instruction in the four major yoga schools (Raja Yoga, Jnana Yoga, Karma Yoga, and Bhakti Yoga). Methods to control the senses, such as trataka (eye exercises) are also important for this kosha. The mind-body practices mentioned earlier help empower people to improve self-control and make the changes necessary to move from unhealthy to healthy habits and lifestyles. This is what yoga therapy for the manomaya kosha does.

Now I will introduce some references from ancient scriptures that are comparable to clinical psychology. Yoga therapists provide counseling with this kind of theoretical background to enable clients to gain self-control over the manomaya kosha.

———

REFERENCE 6: *YOGA SUTRAS* OF PATANJALI
Techniques for Controlling the Senses

Chapter 2 Verse 50

(Pranayama is in) external, internal, or suppressed modification; is regulated by place, time, and number, (and becomes progressively) prolonged and subtle.

Commentary: There are more than one hundred types of pranayama, and they involve a combination of exhalation, inhalation, and breath retention. These are the three "modifications" mentioned in this verse (external, internal, and suppression).

I learned many methods from my guru when I studied under him in the Himalayas from the 1970s through to the 1980s. Such traditional pranayama practices must not, however, be taught to beginners or to people without yoga experience. Pranayama is essentially a practice where respiration—which usually occurs automatically and is controlled by the autonomic nervous system—is regulated according to the intention of the practitioner.

When there is imbalance in the autonomic nervous system, it is very dangerous to prescribe pranayama without understanding the autonomic imbalance and how pranayama can affect those conditions. Many people already have imbalances in their autonomic nervous system, so trying the kinds of pranayama practiced by yogis in the Himalayas could have serious and damaging repercussions on their health. For an instructor to teach pranayama without sufficient knowledge is similar to a doctor prescribing medicine to a patient without knowing the effect the medicine might have. I imagine there are not many doctors who prescribe medicine this way, but unfortunately, there are many yoga instructors who are teaching yoga techniques such as pranayama without understanding their physiological and psychological effects.

If yoga instructors do not assess students' conditions prior to pranayama instruction, detrimental side effects can be expected. It is most dangerous if the yoga instructor also fails to follow up by monitoring the effects of the practices on the student after instruction. Especially in regard to kumbhaka (breath retention), there is insufficient research on the effects of breath retention on unhealthy practitioners. These are things yoga instructors and yoga practitioners should be well aware of before providing instruction or commencing practice.

Chapter 2 Verse 51

That Pranayama that goes beyond the sphere of internal and external is the fourth (variety).

Commentary: While focusing attention on the breath in traditional pranayama practice, our consciousness goes beyond the range of attention and enters a state of complete absorption. This can happen in other practices as well. Patanjali explains that it is at this point when our consciousness unites with Supreme Pure Consciousness. At the Japan Yoga Therapy Society, we adapt traditional pranayama practices, utilizing the psychological changes that pranayama brings forth. We have had success doing this for people with psychosomatic disorders and those who are overadaptive. We have also seen good results using these techniques with schizophrenia patients who are suffering from auditory and visual hallucinations. We use the same theoretical base for yoga therapy for people with drug and other addictions, and are seeing good results in this area too. JYTS prints a compilation of case studies with this evidence every year.

Chapter 2 Verse 33

When the mind is disturbed by improper thoughts, constant pondering over the opposites (is the remedy).

Commentary: The buddhi is one of four psychological organs. In the human chariot theory, the buddhi is the charioteer, holding the reins (manas) by which it receives sensory information about the outside world from the organs of perception (seeing, hearing, tasting, touching, smelling) and organs of action (holding, locomotion, reproduction, elimination, and speech). Based on information the buddhi receives, it understands, predicts, decides, and issues orders for action. It sends those instructions to the manas (reins). It does this repeatedly. After receiving orders from the buddhi through the manas, the organs of perception and action (ten horses) start to work. This is the way traditional yoga explains the way we process outside information.

Traditional yoga also explains how memory is involved. The chitta—the storehouse of memory—sends information from memories to the buddhi, and memories are processed when it does so. Memories stimulate the buddhi, and this information is also sent through the manas to the indriya, the organs of perception and action. Some of this information includes "improper thoughts" that have potentially damaging impacts on the body and can create discord with society. To overcome this, the *Yoga Sutras* provide a method called *pratipaksha bhavanam* ("pondering over opposites"), which involves pulling information from the chitta that counters unhealthy and erroneous thoughts in a way that neutralizes them. It is a kind of psychotherapy that you can also do by yourself. It is necessary for yoga therapists to assess the ability of the client to do this when choosing the yoga techniques to use for clients trying to prevent or overcome lifestyle diseases.

Chapter 2 Verse 52

From that is dissolved the covering of light.

Commentary: In this verse, "from that" is referring to the fourth variety of pranayama mentioned in verse 51 that goes beyond the three modifications of exhalation, inhalation, and retention. "The covering" is a reference to avidya, or ignorance, and "light" refers to wisdom. In other words, from the experience of pure prana, ignorance is dissolved and wisdom is attained.

Whether looking at the pancha kosha theory or the human chariot theory, the foundation of the human structure is the true Self/life principle, the foundation of human existence. According to traditional yoga, the power of life emerges from this principle, and it is the source of divine wisdom and joy. One does not have to be a Nobel laureate to have experienced moments of insight and inspiration that seem to arise from somewhere deep within. This verse is saying that pranayama facilitates such insight and inspiration, and we use this principle in yoga therapy as well.

Chapter 2 Verse 53

And the fitness of the mind for concentration.

Commentary: The fourth variety of pranayama helps to dispel ignorance (verse 52), and also makes the mind ready for the practice of dharana, or concentration. Pranayama is a practice in controlling a function that usually occurs unconsciously, so it requires great focus, even if it is not used for insight. It requires concentration on one thing—breathing according to a specific technique. It is for this reason that pranayama is helpful for people with overadaptive tendencies, as they tend to be easily distracted by other people's opinions and lose sight of themselves. In this sense, pranayama is a useful psychoeducation technique in self-control and stress management.

Chapter 2 Verse 54

Pratyahara, or abstraction is, as it were, the limitation by the senses of the mind by withdrawing themselves from their objects.

Commentary: When completely absorbed in pranayama practice, you can reach the innermost kosha, the anandamaya kosha. At such times, there is no longer awareness of the other koshas. Your consciousness goes deep to the innermost anandamaya kosha and merges with the functions of the chitta, the storehouse of memories. At these times, the functions of the ten sense organs that collect information from the outside world are completely cut off, and this is the complete state of pratyahara, as explained in this verse.

Chapter 2 Verse 55

Then follows the greatest mastery over the senses.

Commentary: Verses 50–55 explain that when we master control of the breath, we also master our sense organs and gain the power of concentration (dharana). In pranayama, we are voluntarily controlling our breathing, which is usually an involuntary function, so the repeated practice of concentrating on voluntarily regulating the breath cultivates our ability to be aware of information from the sense organs, our feelings of likes and dislikes, and so on. Pranayama practice thus cultivates our ability to control the chitta and manas. By assessing these abilities in the client, yoga therapists are effectively providing the most suitable yoga therapy techniques to patients with addiction or mental illnesses, in cooperation with medical professionals.

In the teachings of traditional yoga and Ayurveda, the ten sense organs are said to be the main disturbances, or what causes us humans the most grief. Research in conventional and psychosomatic medicine also shows us that functions of our physical organs, as well as endocrine and immune systems, can be disrupted when the sense organs do not function correctly. Pranayama is effective for regulating the functions of the manomaya kosha, but if practiced incorrectly, it can cause serious adverse events. In my own many years of teaching experience, I have seen students who practiced many more repetitions than they had been instructed and ignored the warnings of their teachers. Over a period of months or years, they developed health problems so severe that they could no longer lead normal lives. If you are interested in pranayama, please make sure that you study under the guidance of a qualified and knowledgeable teacher and follow instructions carefully.

---

4) Prevention of Adverse Events in the Manomaya Kosha

In regard to controlling the ten sense organs, what a person finds enjoyable is largely a matter of personal preference, so it is important for therapists not to judge in terms of good or bad. It is important to work slowly so that clients themselves can adjust their tastes over time in a way that is best for their health. In particular, the organs of perception and action are related to appetite, sex, and material desires, so it is important that therapists do not impose their own values in efforts to change the client's values or preferences.

5) How Changes in the Manomaya Kosha Can Manifest as Physiological Changes

I will now introduce research that shows physiological changes resulting from meditation. Remember, meditation is a practice that is useful in taming the wild horses (sense organs) of the manomaya kosha. The impacts of meditation practice can be seen not only in changes in behavior, but also physical and physiological changes.

A. Meditation Experience Associated with Increased Cortical Thickness

A paper entitled, "Meditation Experience is Associated with Increased Cortical Thickness,"[46] reports on a study comparing the cortical thickness of twenty experienced meditators with a matched control group. Magnetic Resonance Imaging (MRI) was used to measure cortical thickness, and it was found that in comparison to the control group of people without meditation experience, the right anterior insula (associated with attention, interoception, and sensory processing) was thicker in the meditation group. Among the older participants, the difference was very large, indicating that it is possible that meditation can prevent the prefrontal cortex from shrinking with age.

B. Meditation and Prayer Might Change Gene Expression

In 2008, Herbert Benson and his colleagues published a paper entitled, "Genomic Counter-stress Changes Induced by the Relaxation Response" in the July 2 edition of the online journal, *PLoS One.*[47]

Dr. Benson is a pioneer in the field of mind-body medicine, and he first described the relaxation response (opposite of the stress response)

---

46 S. W. Lazar et al., "Meditation Experience is Associated with Increased Cortical Thickness, *Neuroreport* 16, no. 17 (2005): 1893–97.

47 J. A. Dusek et al., "Genomic Counter-Stress Changes Induced by the Relaxation Response," *PLoS ONE* 3 no. 7 (2008): e2576, doi:10.1371/journal.pone.0002576.

thirty-five years ago. Mind-body approaches that elicit the response include a variety of disciplines and methods, including meditation, repetitive prayer, yoga, tai chi, breathing exercises, progressive muscle relaxation, biofeedback, guided imagery, and Qi Gong. According to Dr. Benson, eliciting the relaxation response is useful in treating many ailments, including pain, infertility, rheumatoid arthritis, and insomnia.

In this research, gene expression patterns were compared among nineteen long-time practitioners of a relaxation practice, nineteen healthy controls, and twenty beginners who were given eight weeks of training in a relaxation-response practice. Research results showed that 2,200 genes of long-time practitioners were activated differently in comparison to the control group, and 1,541 genes activated differently in comparison to the beginners' group. Among long-time practitioners and beginners, 433 genes were shared. This indicates that relaxation techniques used in yoga have the potential to turn gene expression on and off. Ayurveda has expounded the psychosomatic and healing benefits of Yoga's breathing and meditation practices since ancient times, and it is now known that this is effective at the genetic level.

C. MEDITATION AND MELATONIN

In the study "Meditation, Melatonin, and Breast/Prostate Cancer: Hypothesis and Preliminary Data,"[48] melatonin levels in urine samples of eight women who meditated regularly were compared with those of eight women who did not meditate. The researchers hypothesized that regular mindfulness meditation practice was related to increased physiological levels of melatonin, and their research indicated that their hypothesis could be correct.

---

48 A. O. Massion et al., "Meditation, Melatonin and Breast/Prostate Cancer: Hypothesis and Preliminary Data," [abstract], Medical Hypotheses 44, no. 1 (1995): 39–46.

6) Fictional Case Studies: Manomaya Kosha

In this section, I will introduce two case studies. As in previous chapters, each case study is a compilation of several actual cases compiled for educational purposes. The case studies in this chapter relate to the manomaya kosha, in which the manas transfers information between the ten indriya (sense organs) and the buddhi (intellect). I hope that this will give you an idea of how yoga therapy works in clinical settings.

Fictional Case Study 5: Yoga Therapy for Depression
(Adapted for Educational Purposes)

1. **Introduction**

    Depression is a common illness in modern society. This is a case study of a hard-working and mild-mannered woman. People around her had high expectations of her. Just before turning sixty, she became ill and had troubles in daily life. She regained her well-being after practicing yoga therapy.

2. **Client Information**

    Physical Information: Female, Age 59 years, Height 157 cm, Weight 56 kg.

    Occupation: Housewife.

    Major Complaints: Anxiety, sense of despair, sleeplessness, depression.

    Family Medical History: Father died from stomach cancer (age 53 years).

    Diagnosis: Anxiety neurosis in year X - 4 (age 55 years) at Mental Hospital A by Psychotherapist B; depression in Year X - 1 (age 58 years) at Mental Hospital C by Psychotherapist D.

    Past Health Problems: Diagnosed with duodenal ulcer in Year X - 7 (age 52 years) by Doctor F at Clinic E and hospitalized for two weeks. Hospitalized again for one month in year X - 2 (age 57 years) in Hospital G.

History of Current Health Problems: She was consistently the top sales woman at an insurance company and had thirty people working under her. She tried to be perfect both at work and at home. In year X - 4 (age 55 years), she went to Mental Clinic A and received medication. It was around that time she began feeling anxiety and lack of motivation. On her days off, even if she was not well, she would do housework and then return to bed. Her family recommended that she quit her job. One day after work, she was unable to prepare dinner. Even while looking at ingredients, she could not think of what to cook and began feeling unexplainable anxiety. In year X - 2 (age 57 years), she had to resign from her job of twenty-four years. Her husband had already retired in year X - 2 (age 57 years). She was unable to get used to the daily rhythm of spending every day with her husband and felt stress about this as well. In year X - 1 (age 58 years), she was diagnosed by Doctor D at Hospital C with depression and began taking medication. In October of year X (age 59 years), she began yoga therapy at the recommendation of her daughter.

Upbringing/Life Circumstances: Raised in a family of five children (one older sister, three older brothers). At thirty-three years of age, her husband (age 36 years) developed lung cancer and had one lung removed. Concerned about the family's future after her husband's illness, she began working at her mother's suggestion. While her husband was in the hospital, one of her older brothers was killed in a farm-tractor accident. A few days after her husband was released from the hospital, her oldest son was hit by a car. After her older brother's death, her mother died of depression at the age of eighty years.

Yoga Therapy History/Changes in Symptoms: She began yoga therapy ninety minutes once a week at a community center in October year X (age 59 years). She explained her diagnosis during the intake, and after obtaining her informed consent to use yoga therapy to address her complaints, we did a more thorough assessment. Her YGPI indicated an unhealthy condition with the following scores: depression 16/20, change of mood 11/20, sense of inferiority 10/20, sensitivity 7/20. Regarding positive characteristics, she scored activity 5/20, mental extroversion 11/20, and social extroversion 15/20. Her personality type was classified as D (directory type), but was marked with emotional instability. On the sVYASA General Health Questionnaire, she scored 7/21 for physical health, 8/21 emotional health, 8/21 social health, and 5/21 spiritual health, totaling 28 of 84 points, putting her in the unhealthy bracket. Her STAI scores showed state anxiety of 50 (stage IV) and trait anxiety 34 (stage III). We also used the SSIM-YSSMA (Yoga Sutra-based State of Mind Assessment), and she scored 4/5 for both number 6 (excessive indulgence) and number 9 (inability to achieve higher levels). The reason for this state of mind was assessed using the SSIM-BGAK (Bhagavad Gita-based Assessment of Karma), in which the score for D (finite/infinite) was a low 2/5 points. At beginning we started her with breathing exercises as yoga therapy, but she could not concentrate well. We began counseling and she was able to talk about her life history. With this counseling, we assessed that she had imbalance in the anandamaya kosha due to the death of her family members. On the APDA, she scored tamas 125/150, rajas 95/150, and sattva 85/150. Tamas was predominant during her intake. We instructed her with isometric sukshma vyayama. On the first day of practice, she was able to feel the condition of her body. We advised that she write a diary, which she did. From January to February of year X + 1 (age 60 years), relatives whose house burned down came to stay at her house. The change in circumstances and perspective may have led to another change seen around May of year X + 1 (age 60 years). Her expression became cheerful and her feelings of pessimism and depression disappeared. While there were fluctuations in her symptoms of insomnia and waking up very early, she was no longer prescribed sleeping pills after September of year X + 1 (age 60 years). At this time, we conducted the SSIM-YSSMA again, and scores for number 6 (excessive indulgence) and number 9 (inability to achieve higher levels) decreased to 2/5 points. Her APDA tamas score decreased to 90/150, rajas to 85/150, and sattva increased to 100/150. Comparing her YGPI scores from September of year X and May of X + 1 (age 60 years), the following improvements in mental stability factors were seen. Her depression score improved from 16 to 0/20, change of mood from 11 to 1/20, sense of inferiority from 10 to 1/20, and sensitivity from 7 to 0/20. For positive characteristics, activity improved from 6 to 13/20, mental extroversion from 11 to 20/20, and social extroversion from 15 to 18/20. Her personality type was director type both times, but the detailed content showed great improvement. The sVYASA General Health Questionnaire showed the following changes between September year X and May year X + 1 (age 60 years). Her physical health improved from 7 to 15/21, emotional health from 8 to 15/21, social health from 8 to 11/21 points, spiritual health from 5 to 18/21 points, making a total score change from 28 to 59 points, indicating good health. In September of year X + 3 (age 62 years), her STAI trait scores were anxiety 33 (stage II) and state anxiety 32 (stage III), indicating she had completely overcome depression. To assess the reasons for some of these changes, we used the SSIM-BGAK, and her score for D (finite/infinite) increased from 2 to 4/5 points.

Client Testimony: I think I've become more flexible. I only take two kinds of medicines now. When I stopped taking sleeping pills, I felt a little uneasy, but my son-in-law said, "losing a little sleep won't kill you." A few days after I heard this, I got used to it, and was OK. I don't vacuum everyday anymore, but only when necessary. My husband helps me prepare for dinner. He shows more understanding to me these days. Before, he did not like women to go to work, but he has acknowledged that we can manage because I have an income. My regular doctor, Doctor D of Hospital C told me in May of year X + 1 (age 60 years) that the way I walked and my facial expressions had changed. These days, when I wait in the waiting room at the hospital, I feel uncomfortable remembering how I used to be. I started to learn the piano (September year X + 1, age 60 years).

3. Observations

This practitioner became exhausted both physically and mentally after years of excessive tension. By practicing yoga therapy, she became more objective. She also experienced entering a new stage in life of retirement with her husband, learning to overcome friction and showing consideration for each other. We advised that she write a diary, which she did. She began to notice her own breathing, bodily sensations, and mental states, which she had never felt before practicing yoga therapy, and she is gradually returning to her true self. All the clinical psychology tests and SSIMs reflected this improvement. In particular, she recovered the ability of discriminate between finite and infinite. These changes in her character helped her recovery. We want to continue working with her to facilitate her full recovery and ability to feel happiness.

Fictional Case Study 6: Yoga Therapy for Premenstrual Syndrome (PMS)

1. Introduction

Premenstrual syndrome (PMS) has a wide variety of symptoms, including mood swings, tender breasts, food cravings, fatigue, irritability, and depression. Symptoms tend to recur in a predictable pattern about two weeks before menstruation. In this case study, the client's symptoms improved after practicing yoga therapy.

2. Client Information

Physical information: Female, Age 31 years, Height 159 cm, Weight 47 kg.

Occupation: Part-time office worker.

Major Complaints: Emotional instability before menstruation; coldness of the lower half of her legs; stiff shoulders and fatigue.

Family History: Father: stomach cancer (age 68 years); Mother: nasal inflammation (age 30 years).

Diagnosis: PMS at year X - 6 (age 25 years). Hospital A, Doctor B.

Past Health Problems: Nasal allergy (age 13 years).

History of Current Health Problems: In year X - 9 (age 22 years), she started work at company A as an accounting clerk, after which she would become emotionally unstable before menstruation. Her periods were heavy and severely painful, sometimes preventing her from going to work. In year X - 8 (age 23 years) she had nasal inflammation, insomnia, and lost mental balance before menstruation. At year X - 6 (age 25 years) she started to care for her father at home and became depressed. After that she took Chinese herbal medicine for half a year, her symptoms were alleviated. In year X - 5 (age 26 years) she found another job, but the major complaints gradually worsened. She tried several therapies, but to no effect. In April year X (age 31 years), she had severe emotional instability before menstruation and two days after starting menstruation she would be bedridden and unable to go to her office. Her mother recommended she practice yoga therapy.

Upbringing/Life Circumstances: She was raised in a family of five children. She lived comfortably, but was weak and sometimes developed fever. At school she sometimes had to skip physical education classes. She tended to think too much and was nervous. When she was fifteen, her family moved, and she could not get used to her new circumstances and felt mentally and physically unbalanced for a year. At twenty-two, she graduated college and started to work at an office. Now at thirty-one, she is living with her boyfriend.

Yoga Therapy History/Changes in Symptoms: From April to September year X (age 31 years), she practiced yoga therapy 90 to 120 minutes once or twice a week (total of eight times) at her home. During the first intake, she provided the name of her diagnosis and her major complaints. After obtaining her informed consent to address her complaints, we asked her to take the STAI test in which trait anxiety marked 47 (stage IV high degree) and state anxiety marked 43 (stage IV). On the sVYASA General Health Questionnaire, she had the following low scores of A (physical health) 7/21, B (emotional health) 10/21, C (social health) 10/21, and D (spiritual health) 7/21 to total 34/84 points, indicating an unhealthy condition.

Furthermore, she complained about her work and of anxiety about her health. From her mental tendencies and current health history, we assessed that she was very sensitive and serious, had a tendency to overadapt, set high standards for herself, and was looking for acceptance from others. Unable to meet her own standards, she was very harsh on herself. By this yogic assessment and considering other psychological tests we assessed her mental condition using the SSIM-YSSMA (Yoga Sutra-based State of Mind Assessment), and she scored 5/5 for number 6 (excessive indulgence) and number 9 (inability to achieve higher levels), indicating an unhealthy mental condition. The reason for this state of mind was assessed using the SSIM-YSAM (Yoga Sutra-based Assessment of Misrecognition) in which the score for D (misrecognition of "not Self" as "Self") was the highest 5/5 points. We concluded our assessment that the defects in manomaya and vijnanamaya koshas were the main causes of her major complaints.

Using the SSIM-AISO (Assessment of Intellectual-Sensibility and Objectivity) for her mental assessment, we found that number 5 (ability to act—order and objectivity) marked a low 2/5. She was unable to notice when she became caught up in oversensitive reactions to unpleasant conditions. Her breath had become habitually fast and shallow, and she was physically stiff, all indications of imbalances in her annamaya, pranamaya, and manomaya koshas.

To cultivate her objective awareness, we first instructed her in breathing exercises and sukshma vyayama, asanas, quick-relaxation technique, deep-relaxation technique, and some kinds of pranayama. In the beginning she could not close her eyes because of strong anxiety. From May of year X (age 31 years), we introduced isometric resistance into her yoga therapy practice. We monitored the changes in her condition and noticed better concentration, and she reported feeling warmth around her waist and feeling calmer. Then she started practicing on her own at home. But in July of year X (age 31 years), she expressed feeling obligated to practice and some obsessiveness toward the results of her practice.

Before she started this yoga therapy practice, she had tried several other therapies. Considering this tendency, we assessed her character using the SSIM-BGAK (Bhagavad Gita-based Assessment of Karma), in which her score for A (ability to see beyond polarity) was a low 2/5 and her intellect sheath was out of balance. So we started with the verbal counseling and instructed her to focus on the present through Karma Yoga, and to practice asana without worrying too much about how many repetitions or types she practiced.

In August of year X (age 31 years), she showed improved awareness of her breath and physical condition in daily life. She also started to enjoy the yoga therapy class, and she overcame the shoulder stiffness and fatigue. She spoke less negatively. It was clear her behavior was changing and the function of her vijnanamaya kosha improved gradually. To monitor the changes in her condition, she took the STAI and sVYASA self-health test. sVYASA self-health test showed the following changes between September year X and May year X + 1. Physical health improved from 7 to 15/21, emotional health from 10 to 15/21, social health from 10 to 18/21 points, and spiritual health from 7 to 18/21 points, making a total score change from 34 to 64/84 points. In September of year X + 3, her STAI trait scores improved (anxiety from 47 to 33 (stage II) and state anxiety 43 to 32 (stage III), indicating she had completely overcome depression.

In September year X (age 31 years) her shoulder stiffness and fatigue reduced. The coldness in her lower legs showed no improvement, but she felt warmth after practice and was no longer concerned about it. Her SSIM-YSSMA scores for number 6 (excessive indulgence) and number 9 (inability to achieve) improved from 5/5 to 2/5 points. Her expression brightened and she seemed more mentally stable. At this time, we assessed SSIM-BGAK, in which her score for A (ability to see beyond polarity) increased from 2/5 to 4/5 points and her mental assessment based on the SSIM-AISO indicated that number 5 (ability to act—order and objectivity) increased from 2/5 to 4/5 points. We concluded our assessment that the functions of all koshas, from manomaya to anandamaya, had improved.

Client Testimony: By continuing yoga therapy, I was able to feel the condition of my body in ways I could not before. I don't get stuck in negativity as much. I want to become strong enough to maintain my sense of well-being.

3. Observations

By repeatedly practicing awareness of both physical and mental changes through yoga therapy practice, this practitioner was able to develop her capacity to observe herself. Previous imbalances in her vijnanamaya kosha had triggered various symptoms, but her sensitivity began to work in a more positive direction, without showing the same hypersensitivity she had displayed previously. Her sVYASA self-health test showed improvement, and was consistent with improvements in her STAI, SSIM-YSSMA, SSIM-YSAM, SSIM-AISO, and SSIM-BGAK scores. By continuing her own practice at home, she noticed her ability to control

Yoga Therapy Theory

symptoms and emotions, and gained confidence. This is reflected in the more positive attitudes seen in the clinical psychology and SSIM test results.

CHAPTER 4

Yoga Therapy Assessment (YTA) and Yoga Therapy Instruction (YTI) For The Vijnanamaya Kosha: Addressing Functions of the Buddhi and Forgotten Memories

1) YOGA THERAPY'S PATHOGENESIS THEORY AND THE VIJNANAMAYA KOSHA

OUR BODIES HAVE VARIOUS ORGANS, such as the heart, lungs, and liver. Traditional yoga says we also have four psychological organs, one of them being the buddhi. From a western psychological perspective, the buddhi can be understood as intellect or sensibility. Its characteristic function is to recognize the information from the ten horses (organs of perception and action) and then to discern, predict, decide, and issue orders for action. The orders for action are sent to another psychological organ, the manas (the mind/reins), which then guides five organs of perception (eyes, ears, etc.) and five organs of action (hands, feet, etc.) which then start moving accordingly.

From a yoga therapy perspective, unhealthy functions by the organs of perception and action arise when the buddhi's functions of recognition and discernment are compromised, often leading to stress-related disorders, include psychosomatic illnesses and lifestyle diseases. The problems in the buddhi create effects that ripple to the physical body. For example, breathing changes after misapprehension of an outside stimulus by the buddhi. The hypothalamus controls the body's respiratory functions, and when it is affected, other functions of the autonomic nervous system are also influenced, potentially leading to problems in cardiorespiratory functions and disrupted breathing.

Illnesses that arise due to mistaken cognition have been understood in Ayurveda as imbalances in the psychological doshas (rajas and tamas), and can cause many disorders, such as neurosis, adaptation disorder, and psychosomatic diseases. This mistaken cognition, or misapprehension of information from the ten indriyas by the vijnanamaya kosha, is called "ignorance" in yoga. Ignorance includes, for example, mistaking what is finite for the infinite, or harboring negative feelings such as stubbornness, obsession, anxiety, and depression. There is also ignorance in the way the vijnanamaya kosha apprehends information from memories stored in the chitta (an organ of the anandamaya kosha).

2) Yoga Therapy Assessment (YTA) and the Vijnanamaya Kosha

A. Assessment Using Tools from Psychosomatic Medicine

Questionnaires used in psychosomatic medicine can be used to assess alexisomia,[49] alexithymia,[50] and overadaptation. One example is the Toronto Alexithymia Scale (TAS-20). Yoga therapists should inquire with experts in psychosomatic medicine before using these questionnaires.

B. Assess Intellect, Sensitivity, and Objectivity

Yoga therapists can assess the functions of the buddhi (recognition, discrimination, prediction, decision-making, and the ability to issue orders)

---

49 The condition of having difficulty in experiencing bodily feelings.
50 Difficulty in experiencing, expressing, and describing emotional responses.

by using the *Semi-Structured Interview Manual-Assessment of Intellectual-Sensibility and Objectivity* (SSIM-AISO).

C. Assess Ability to Control Sense Organs

Yoga therapists can use the *Semi-Structured Interview Manual-Assessment of the Indriyas* (SSIM-AI) to assess the client's capacity to regulate organs of perception and action.

D. Use Inventories from Clinical Psychology

To assess clients' mental states, yoga therapists can use inventories from clinical psychology such as the YGPI, sVYASA General Health Questionnaire, POMS, and STAI.

E. Assess Cognitive Functions

Yoga therapists should assess clients' standards of cognition. To do so, they can use the SSIM-YSSMA and the SSIM-YSAM. The *Yoga Sutras* of Patanjali provide various methods to assess the human mind and standards for ideal mental conditions and mentality. This is basically equivalent to mental physiology, and the verses I will introduce next provide us with a standard by which to measure healthy psychological functions.

———

REFERENCE 7: VERSES FROM CHAPTER 1 OF THE *YOGA SUTRAS*

Chapter 1 Verse 30

Disease, languor, doubt, carelessness, laziness, worldly minded-ness, delusion, nonachievement of a stage, instability, these (nine) cause the distraction of the mind and they are the obstacles.

Chapter 1 Verse 31

(Mental) pain, despair, nervousness, and hard breathing are the symptoms of a distracted condition of mind.

Commentary: Patanjali compiled teachings that had been traditionally passed down by generations of yogis into the *Yoga Sutras*. He mentions nine kinds of mental disturbances as obstacles to samadhi. For the ancient yogis who were striving to attain samadhi, such mental disturbances were the greatest obstacles and needed to be addressed, so they would analyze their own minds, find the causes of disturbance and eliminate them. In our modern times, we can do the same. It is especially important for yoga therapists to do so themselves, in order to guide clients as effectively as possible. With purified minds, yoga therapists can utilize their own experiences to understand their clients and to assess mental weaknesses in accordance with the nine obstacles mentioned by Patanjali.

REFERENCE 8: YOGA SUTRA VERSE CHAPTER 2 VERSE 5

Avidya is taking the noneternal, impure, evil and non-Atman to be eternal, pure, good and Atman, respectively.

Commentary: Avidya is often translated as "ignorance." In *Yoga Sutras* Verse 2.3, Patanjali explains the causes of life's miseries to be, "ignorance, the sense of egoism or 'I-am-ness,' attachment, aversion, and desire for life." In Verse 2.4, he goes on to explain that ignorance is also the source of the other causes mentioned in the same verse. This is the case "whether they be in the dormant, attenuated, alternating, or expanded condition."

It is after this that he explains ignorance as mistaking something for what it is not, that is, mistaking noneternal for eternal, impure for pure, evil for good, and non-*Atman* for *Atman*. Patanjali also provides methods to remove these obstacles, one being Verse 1.32, that is, "[f]or removing these obstacles, there (should be) constant practice of one truth or principle."

———

As seen in references 7 and 8, traditional yoga provides standards to assess imbalances in the mind, explanations for their causes, and methods to overcome them. Yoga therapy takes traditional yoga's techniques and adapts them based on yoga's "physiology of the human mind" so that they can be used to address stress-related illnesses in the context of our modern society.

F. ASSESS ACTION/KARMA

Yoga therapists also assess clients' abilities of action/Karma. For this assessment, yoga therapists can use the SSIM-BGAK (Bhagavad Gita-based Assessment of Karma). In this assessment, yoga therapists assess the following factors: A—ability to see beyond polarity; B—control of the five sense organs; C—concentration; and D—distinguishing between finite and infinite. Using these assessments, yoga therapists can assess clients' lifestyles and create programs to address imbalances. I will explain these four factors, A through D, as they appear in the *Bhagavad Gita*. In this way, yoga therapy uses the teachings of ancient scriptures for assessment of clients' body-mind conditions.

A—Ability to See Beyond Polarity

Bhagavad Gita Chapter 2: *Sankhya Yoga* Verse 38

Having made pleasure and pain, gain and loss, victory and defeat the same, engage thou in battle for the sake of battle; thus thou shalt not incur sin.

Commentary: Our worldly lives are filled with dualities such as pleasure and pain, loss, and gain. Our emotions are also often disturbed by those dualities, or we may feel caught between them. It is possible, however, to transcend duality to maintain equanimity.

In Japan, we have a saying that "everything in life is like the story of the farmer and his horse." It is a saying based on a story from ancient China about a farmer whose horse runs away. Neighbors lament, but the farmer does not. The horse returns with a stallion. The neighbors call it a blessing until the farmer's son tries to ride it and is kicked off and crippled as a result of the injury. The neighbors think it is a curse, until war breaks out and the son is not enlisted. He continues to live at home while lives of other young men are lost in battle. Throughout it all, the farmer maintains equanimity.

This saying has been translated into English as, "inscrutable are the ways of heaven." It tells us that we can never really know whether a given situation is good or bad. It is therefore best to accept the situation first, and then consider how to handle it, without losing equanimity by getting lost in the ideas of whether the situation is a blessing or bane. This is also what the *Bhagavad Gita* is teaching when Lord Krishna orders Arjuna to prepare for war. Yoga therapists need to assess to what degree clients have this kind of mindset, because without it, clients will experience much undue stress.

B—Control of the Five Sense Organs

Bhagavad Gita Chapter 2: *Sankhya Yoga* Verse 58

When, like the tortoise which withdraws its limbs on all sides, he withdraws his senses from the sense-objects, then his wisdom becomes steady.

Commentary: In Ayurvedic pathogenesis and in traditional yoga, the root of all mental disturbances is in the relationship between senses and sense-objects. According to the human chariot theory, we can live healthy lives if the buddhi (charioteer/intellect) can skillfully control the ten indriyas (horses/organs of perception and action). For that purpose, it is important that the horses do not run in wild pursuit of worldly things including food, shelter, and clothing. It is like "the tortoise which withdraws its limbs on all sides." This does not mean that food, shelter, and clothing need to be rejected. It simply means that being overly attached to or distracted by the objects of the senses leads to suffering. It is important that yoga therapists be able to assess the degree to which clients can control their attachment to objects of the senses.

Bhagavad Gita Chapter 2: *Sankhya Yoga* Verse 62

When a man thinks of the objects, attachment to them arises; from attachment desire is born; from desire anger arises.

Commentary: This verse explains the mechanism for the onset of desire and anger, which are among the causes of psychological disorders. The stronger we want to obtain the objects of our senses, which begin with food, clothing and shelter, the more upset we get when our desires are not fulfilled. It is necessary for yoga therapists to assess the degree these negative feelings of rajas and tamas are predominant in the mind. Based on the assessments, therapists should guide clients so that the clients themselves can become aware of their own negativity and overcome it through yoga therapy.

C—Concentration

Bhagavad Gita Chapter 3: Selfless Action Verse 8

Do thou perform thy bounden duty, for action is superior to inaction and even the maintenance of the body would not be possible for thee by inaction.

Commentary: Each one of us has various duties depending on our situation. We have our positions in our families, workplaces, and among friends and acquaintances. If we focus on performing the duties that come with our position, we will be evaluated highly by those around us. If we are not able to perform our duties, regardless of the reason, we of course gain a reputation for not fulfilling our responsibilities. Before talking about whether or not we have the ability to fulfill duties, the question is whether or not we are able to concentrate well enough to perform them. It is important for yoga therapists to assess whether clients have sufficient capacity in concentration.

Bhagavad Gita Chapter 4: Liberation from Action Verse 10

Freed from attachment, fear and anger, absorbed in Me, taking refuge in Me, purified by the fire of knowledge, many have attained to My Being.

Commentary: Attachment, fear, and anger exacerbate our mental doshas. Yoga therapists need to assess the client for prevalence in these feelings, and then help clients recognize their own feelings. Therapists also provide instruction based on yoga's traditional teachings so that clients can be "purified by the fire of knowledge."

D—Ability to Distinguish Finite from Infinite

Bhagavad Gita Chapter 9: The King of Knowledge, King of Secrets Verse 11

Fools disregard Me, clad in human form, not knowing My higher Being as the great Lord of (all) beings.

Commentary: As we saw in the story of the farmer and his horse, it is better to accept what happens without resisting what we cannot change. Inscrutable are the ways of heaven. This way of thinking, however, should not be forced upon clients, as people have different faiths and personal beliefs. In life, however, we will always encounter events that are beyond human control and understanding, be it daily changes in the weather or large natural disasters. When we find ourselves faced with such events, no amount of complaining or insisting that we have done nothing wrong and do not deserve such things will bring about a solution. It is best to maintain a stable mind and respond to the situation at hand. Yoga therapists need to assess whether clients have this capacity, and then based on the assessment, determine what kinds of yoga techniques are best.

Bhagavad Gita Chapter 11: The Vision of Cosmic Person Verse 49

Be not afraid nor bewildered on seeing such a terrible form of Mine as this; with thy fear entirely dispelled and with a gladdened heart, now behold again this former form of Mine.

Commentary: In previous verses, Arjuna requests Lord Krishna to reveal God in all of God's glory. Krishna warns him that the sight of God is not easy to behold, and shows his pure form. Arjuna is nearly overwhelmed by the sight, but the Lord tells Arjuna not to be afraid, explaining in this verse that everything that Arjuna beholds is a manifestation of God.

The "ways of heaven" do not necessarily match what we think is most convenient or best. For example, earthquakes, massive floods, and typhoons, as well as economic change and other social changes may not happen in the ways we expect or hope. Some things seem clearly divine, such as breathtaking scenery and people of incredible kindness or talent. But there are also people who commit atrocities that can only be thought of as evil. What this verse teaches us is that all are manifestations of God, or "the ways of heaven." The wise always understand that heaven has its way in any matter, and it is with this understanding that they respond to difficult situations and become known for their intelligence. Yoga therapists must develop this quality within themselves, in addition to providing such guidance and education to clients.

REFERENCE 9

The two following inventories are based on the *Bhagavad Gita*. One was made in India, and the other in the United States.

1. Standardization of the *Gita* Inventory of Personality[51]
2. The Vedic Personality Inventory by Dr. David Wolf

G. The Assessment of Mental Doshas in Ayurveda

Here I will introduce some standards for assessment used in Ayurvedic medicine. It is said that each person has an inherent mental constitution (*manas prakrti*) that is determined at the time of conception and does not change throughout the person's lifetime. The mental constitution is determined by the degree of predominance of the three gunas—sattva, rajas, and tamas. I will introduce some verses from the *Charaka Samhita*, but before that, allow me to briefly explain the three mental constitutions, or manas prakrti.

Sattvika Prakrti

When the sattva guna is most predominant in a person's mental constitution, the person is said to have *sattvika prakrti*. Such a person tends to be gentle, tolerant, honest, spiritually healthy, to have a good memory, be imaginative, intellectually creative, brave, and able to share both joy and sorrow with others. Sattvika people are not disturbed by dualities like good and bad, joy and sorrow, and likes and dislikes.

Rajasika Prakrti

When the rajas guna is most predominant, the person is said to have *rajasika prakrti*. A rajasika person is said to be generally a pathological

---

51 R. C. Das, "Standardization of the Gita Inventory of Personality," *Journal of Indian Psychology* 9 nos. 1 and 2 (1991): 47–54.

liar, brutal in nature, conceited, proud, prurient, angry, cowardly, selfish, and has strong likes and dislikes. Rajasika people want to be busy all the time. Charaka explains that rajasika can be divided into six types, as explained later in Reference 11.

Tamasa Prakrti

When the tamas guna is most predominant, a person is said to have *tamasa prakrti*. People of tamasa prakrti have qualities of sadness, atheism, evilness, ignorance, foolishness, lethargy, and prefer to avoid mental and physical activity. Charaka divides tamasa prakrti into three types, as explained in Reference 11.

A person with predominant rajas or tamas qualities has unhealthy mentalities but may not necessarily show physical illness. They are, however, easily affected by stress, anxiety, and depression.

There is a strong connection between the three physical doshas (vata, pitta, and kapha) and the three gunas (sattva, rajas, and tamas). The body and mind are interdependent, and they cannot be separated. One imbalance will trigger another imbalance to some degree, and this is why Ayurveda considers all diseases to be mind-body illnesses. I will now introduce some teachings from the *Charaka Samhita* to illustrate.

REFERENCE 10: MENTAL AND PHYSICAL DOSHAS, FROM THE *CHARAKA SAMHITA*

Charaka Samhita: Vimanasthana Chapter VI Verse 5[52]

> *Because of their highly multitudinous nature, diseases are innumerable. On the other hand, doshas are numerable because of their limitation in number. So only some of the diseases will be explained by way of illustrations, whereas doshas will be explained in their*

---

52 *Caraka Samhita*, vol. II, 186.

entirety. Rajas and tamas are the doshas pertaining to the mind, and the types of morbidity caused by them are passion (kama), anger, greed, attachment, envy, ego, pride, grief, worry, anxiety, fear, excitement, etc. Vata, pitta, and kapha—these three are the doshas pertaining to the body. Diseases caused by them are fever, diarrhea, edema, consumption, dyspnea, meha (obstinate urinary disorder including diabetes), kustha (obstinate skin diseases including leprosy), etc. Thus doshas in their entirety and diseases in parts are explained.

Commentary: Earlier, I explained how in Ayurveda, there are two categories of *doshas*, or causes of disease. One is mental (consisting of rajas and tamas), and the other is physical (consisting of vata, pitta, and kapha). These concepts existed in India thousands of years ago, prior to knowledge of bacteria, and illness was understood to be disturbance of mental and physical balance. These ancient teachings were forgotten for some time, but they are being revived. In spite of the development of modern medicine, we are seeing an increase in disease. This is due to the global increase in stress-related diseases that occur when mental and physical balance is disrupted. I believe that Ayurveda's teachings may be one tool to save the health of our modern society, and yoga therapy techniques are essential as the practices used in Ayurveda to restore people's conditions from rajasic or tamasic states to sattvic states.

Charaka Samhita: Vimanasthana **Chapter VI Verse 8**[53]

When allowed to persist for long, these psychic diseases, viz., kama (passion) etc., and somatic diseases viz., fever etc., at times get combined with each other.

Commentary: It is clear from this verse that Charaka already understood, in 300 BC, that there is a clear relationship between the mind and the body.

---

53 *Caraka Samhita*, vol. II, 187.

Charaka Samhita: Sharira Sthana Chapter IV Verse 34[54]

Now, there are three physical doshas *(vitiating elements), viz., vata, pitta and kapha—they vitiate the body. Again there are two mental* doshas, *viz., rajas and tamas—they vitiate the mind. Vitiation of the body and the mind result in the manifestation of diseases—there is no disease without their vitiation.*

Commentary: In this verse, Charaka is saying that mental *doshas* disrupt physical *doshas*, and this leads to the appearance of disease in the physical body, the annamaya kosha. In Japan, we are seeing increasing numbers of clinics treating patients for a growing epidemic of psychosomatic disorders. I cannot help but think that yoga therapy would be of great assistance to people wanting to restore mind-body balance.

Charaka Samhita: Sharira Sthana Chapter IV Verse 36[55]

Mental faculty is of three types—sattvika, rajasa, and tamasa. Sattvika is free from defects as it is endowed with auspiciousness. Rajasa is defective because it promotes wrathful disposition. Tamasa is similarly defective because it suffers from ignorance.

Each of the three types of mental faculty is in fact of innumerable variety by permutation and combination of the various factors relating to the body, species, and mutual interactions. Sometimes even the body follows the mind and vice versa. So we shall now explain some of the varieties of mental faculties briefly by way of illustration.

Commentary: In Ayurveda, mental conditions are explained in terms of predominance of *gunas*. But even when one guna is predominant, the other gunas are always present to some degree. They never completely

---

54 *Caraka Samhita*, vol. II, 405.
55 *Caraka Samhita*, vol. II, 406.

Yoga Therapy Theory

disappear. Depending on the predominance, there are categories of mental states as explained in verses that follow. All have come from ancient Indian tradition, hence the use of the names of deities and gods.

REFERENCE 11: THE MENTAL DOSHAS IN AYURVEDA: THE IDEAL SATTVIKA AND THE VITIATED RAJASA AND TAMASA

The *Charaka Samhita* includes the following explanation about the mental doshas. Examining the characteristics of sattvika in comparison with rajasa and tamasa, it is clear that sattvika is the most healthy and balanced mental faculty. It is, as explained in this verse, "free from defects as it is endowed with auspiciousness." It therefore provides an explanation of an ideal mental state, which also acts as a standard against which to measure the degree of disease. Rajasa and tamasa mental faculties, as seen in the explanations that follow, contain characteristics that can be identified as potential causes of illness.

Because the descriptions were written in accordance with Indian culture and tradition at the time, there are many expressions that would not likely be used today. It is important to look beyond the names of Indian deities, for example, and to see what it is that the verses are teaching. It is evident that the teachings are very applicable to health issues we are facing in our modern world, and we can easily follow the teachings of Charaka.

Charaka Samhita: Sharira Sthana Chapter IV Verses 37–40
Seven Types of Sattvika[56]

The sattvika type of mental faculty is auspicious and is of seven categories. Their characteristic features are furnished in the statement given below:

1. Brahma: Purity, love for truth, self-controlled; power of discrimination, material and spiritual knowledge; power of exposition, reply, and memory; freedom from passion, anger, greed, ego,

---

56 *Caraka Samhita*, vol. II, 407.

183

ignorance, jealousy, dejection, and intolerance; and favorable disposition equally for all creatures.

2. Arsa: devotion to sacred rituals, study, sacred vows, oblations, and celibacy; hospitable disposition; freedom from pride, ego, attachment, hatred, ignorance, greed and anger; intellectual excellence and eloquence; and power of understanding and retention.
3. Aindra: Lord-ship and authoritative speech; performance of sacred rituals; bravery, strength, and splendor; freedom from mean acts; far sightedness; and devotion to virtuous acts, earning of wealth and proper satisfaction of desires.
4. Yamya: observance of the propriety of actions; initiation of actions in time; nonviolability; readiness for initiating action; memory and lordship; freedom from attachment, envy, hatred, and ignorance.
5. Varuna: bravery, patience, purity, and dislike for impurity; observance of religious rites; fondness for aquatic sports; aversion for mean acts; and exhibition of anger and pleasure in proper place.
6. Kauvera: possession of station, honor, luxuries, and attendants; constant liking for virtuous acts, wealth, and satisfaction of desires, purity; and liking for pleasures of recreation.
7. Gandharva: fondness for dancing, singing, music, and praise; expertness in poetry, stories, historical narrations, and epics; constant fondness for scents, garlands, unguents apparel, association of women, and passion.

Of the seven types of *sattvika* mental faculties described above, the one likened to Brahma is the purest.

Different types of *rajasa* individuals:

The *rajasika* type of mental faculty represents wrathful disposition and is of six types. Their characteristic features are furnished in the statement given below:

1. Asura: bravery, cruelty, envy, lordship, movement in disguise, terrifying appearance and ruthlessness; and indulgence in self-praise.

Yoga Therapy Theory

2. Raksasa: intolerance, constant anger, violence at weak points, cruelty, gluttonous habit, and fondness for nonvegetarian food; excessive sleep and indolence; and envious disposition.
3. Paisaca: gluttonous habit; fondness for women; liking for staying with women in lonely places; unclean habits, disliking for cleanliness; cowardice and terrifying disposition; and resorting to abnormal diet and regimens.
4. Sarpa: bravery when in wrathful disposition and cowardice when not in wrathful disposition; sharp reaction; excessive indolence; and walking, taking food, and resorting to other regimens with a fearful disposition.
5. Praita: excessive desire for food; excessively painful disposition in character and past times; enviousness; and actions without discrimination, excessive greediness, and inaction.
6. Sakuna: attachment with passion, excessive food and regimen, unsteadiness, ruthlessness, and unacquisitiveness.

Different types of tamasa individuals:

1. Pasava: forbidding disposition; lack of intelligence; hateful conduct and food habit; excessive sexual indulgence and sleep.
2. Matsya: cowardice, lack of intelligence, greediness for food, unsteadiness, constant passionate, and wrathful disposition; and fondness for constant movement and desire for water.
3. Vanaspatya: indolence, indulgence in food, and deficiency of all the intellectual faculties.

REFERENCE 12: AYURVEDIC PSYCHOLOGICAL DOSHA ASSESSMENT (APDA)

The Japan Yoga Therapy Society developed an assessment of clients' mental state based on the Ayurvedic doshas. This tool is called the Ayurvedic Psychological Dosha Assessment (APDA).

Following is a chart that shows the different characteristics that belong to each type of mental constitution.

MENTAL CONSTITUTION			
Mental Functions	Sattva	Rajas	Tamas
Concentration	Very clear	Hyperactive	Cloudy
Memory	Good	Moderate	Poor
Will power	Good	Moderate	Poor
Honesty	Very good	Variable	Weak
Peace of mind	Always	Mostly	Rarely
Creativity	Generally	Occasionally	Rarely
Spiritual study	High	Moderate	Low
Mantra/Prayer	Daily	Occasionally	Never
Meditation	Daily	Occasionally	Never
Selfless service	Often	Occasionally	Rarely
Relationships	Harmonious	Passionate	Disturbed
Anger	Rarely	Frequently	Frequently
Fear	Rarely	Sometimes	Frequently
Desire	Little	Some	Uncontrollable
Pride	No ego	Some ego	Egoistic
Depression	Never	Sometimes	Frequently
Love	Universal	Personal	Lacking in love
Violent behavior	Never	Sometimes	Frequently
Attachment	Detached	Occasionally	Attached
Forgiveness	Forgive easily	With effort	Grudges
Diet	Vegetarian	Some meat	Frequent meat

Addictive behavior	Never	Occasionally	Frequently
Sensory impression	Calm	Mixed	Disturbed
Sleep requirement	Little	Moderate	Excessive
Sexual activity	Controlled	Intense	Uncontrollable
Control of senses	Good	Moderate	Low
Speech	Peaceful	Agitated	Dull
Cleanliness	High	Moderate	Low
Work	Selfless	Reward centered	Aimless

3) Principles of Yoga Therapy Instruction (YTI) for the Vijnanamaya Kosha

The aim of yoga therapy for the vijnanamaya kosha is to correct malfunctioning of the buddhi, the charioteer. When clients already have difficulty interacting with society and have problems evident in the annamaya, pranamaya and manomaya koshas, we can assess the vijnanamaya kosha's functions of recognizing incoming information, discerning, predicting, deciding, and giving orders for action. First, clients are instructed in breathing exercises so they can become aware of both body and breathing. In this way, they become gradually more aware of the vijnanamaya kosha's functions and learn to control them. The primary method used is called *samyama*, a type of meditation in Raja Yoga, and it is also a type of Vedic meditation dating from the times of the Upanishads and practiced in the

Himalayas for some four thousand to five thousand years. Raja Yoga meditation is also mentioned in the *Yoga Sutras*, such as in the excerpt from chapter 2 that follows.

Yoga Sutras Chapter 2 Verses 3, 10–12

(3) *The lack of awareness of Reality, the sense of egoism or "I-am-ness," attractions and repulsions toward objects and the strong desire for life are the great afflictions or causes of all miseries in life.*

(10) *These, the subtle ones, can be reduced by resolving them backward into their origin.*

(11) *Their active modifications are to be suppressed by meditation.*

(12) *The reservoir of karmas that are rooted in kleshas brings all kinds of experiences in the present and future lives.*

While guiding clients in meditation techniques, yoga therapists also teach traditional yoga philosophy as psychoeducation in order to give clients a standard for decision-making. Yoga therapists teach these ideal standards for decision-making from the four main schools of yoga—Jnana Yoga, Raja Yoga, Bhakti Yoga, and Karma Yoga. Some verses and teachings used are introduced subsequently.

The four points that follow are a summary of yoga therapy instruction for the vijnanamaya kosha.

- Yoga therapists help clients correct their cognition by observing the way they apprehend and understand their own memories and sensory/intellectual activities.
- Yoga therapists address the vijnanamaya kosha to enable clients to attain both mental and physical self-control. In this way, yoga therapists should try to help clients cultivate not only physical, mental, and social health, but also spiritual health, bringing clients to the state of perfect health (liberation).
- Yoga therapists usually use Raja Yoga meditation and Vedic meditation techniques for this kosha.

* Counseling, psychoeducation, and the four major traditional yoga philosophies are also essential for this kosha.

4) Purification of and Instruction for the Vijnanamaya Kosha

For the vijnanamaya kosha, we use Raja Yoga meditation (explained in Patanjali's *Yoga Sutras*) and Vedic meditation (listening, contemplation, meditation on daily life, realization). Reference 13 introduces the theory and its historical description as written in the scriptures.

———

REFERENCE 13: PATANJALI'S *YOGA SUTRAS*

From Chapter 2 on Raja Yoga Meditation Verse 28

From the practice of the component exercises of Yoga, on the destruction of impurity, arises spiritual illumination, which develops into awareness of Reality.

Commentary: Patanjali explains more about the "component exercises of Yoga" in verse 29. These "component exercises" are more commonly known as the "eight limbs of yoga," and dedicated practice of these eight limbs leads to disappearance of mental impurities. Indeed, verse 43 of chapter 2 makes this clear:

"Perfection of the sense-organs and body after destruction of impurity by austerities."

This means that repeated and dedicated practice of these eight limbs as tapas (austerities) will purify our minds.

In addition, chapter 18 verse 37 of the *Bhagavad Gita* speaks about the repeated practice of meditation as "which in the beginning is like poison (and) when there is transformation, is like nectar, that happiness is called 'sattvika,' born of the clarity of self-knowledge."

Thus, the scriptures tell us that repeated practice of austerities will bring us to destruction of impurity.

Patanjali lists the eight limbs of yoga in Chapter 2 Verse 29:

Self-restraint (yama), fixed observance (niyama), posture (asana), regulation of breath (pranayama), abstraction (pratyahara), concentration (dharana), contemplation (dhyana), (and) trance (samadhi) are the eight parts (of the self-discipline of Yoga).

Commentary:

The eight limbs of the self-discipline of yoga aim to purify the mind. When the mind is purified, pure consciousness, or Self, can manifest untainted, straight through the anandamaya and vijnanamaya koshas, to shine through the outermost sheaths of our being.

The first of the eight limbs of yoga are the yamas, five self-restraints to refrain from violence, untruthfulness, stealing, sexual indulgence, and covetousness. The second limb is the niyamas—that is, purification, contentment, austerity, study of scriptures, and self-surrender. The third limb is asana to train the physical body, and the fourth is pranayama, which is control of the breath. Fifth is pratyahara, controlling the senses, and the sixth is dharana, or concentration. The seventh limb is dhyana, which means meditation, and the last stage is samadhi, or a very deep meditation in which we are led from the anandamaya kosha to realize the Self. We practice these eight limbs of yoga, step by step, to purify our minds, and yoga therapists utilize simplified versions of these Raja Yoga techniques to help clients purify their own minds and overcome disease.

Next, I will introduce the sutras on some of the yamas and niyamas.

Yoga Sutras Chapter 2 Verse 35 on Nonviolence (Ahimsa)

"On being firmly established in nonviolence there is abandonment of hostility in (his/her) presence."

Commentary: From this verse onward, Patanjali explains the social phenomena that occur once the mind is purified. In this verse, he says that when a person no longer has violence in thought, word, or action, that no living creature, let alone other people, will approach with any hostility. This verse teaches us that the violence we experience is a reflection of the violence in our own minds. When our minds contain violence, that violence befalls us as well, so the best way to prevent it is to purify our own minds. We can learn from this sutra to examine our own hearts, minds, and behavior for violence, and see how that may be reflected in the things we experience in everyday life. This verse can also be used as a standard of measure during assessment of clients.

Yoga therapists provide meditation instruction based on these teachings. It is possible, however, that clients may not be ready to hear these things, and trying to teach before they are ready can lead to unnecessary resistance toward the teachings. It is important to assess a client's readiness before deciding what kinds of meditation content and techniques to provide.

Dr. Kent M. Keith's "The Paradoxical Commandments" are a modern example of teachings of ahimsa as well as Karma Yoga. He wrote them for high school students when he was a college student at Harvard University. They encourage us to handle stressful situations by continuing to live according to what we know to be right. Regardless of the varying degrees of violent reactions we may experience from others, if we can develop the inner strength to continue to do what we know to be right, we can maintain our own peace of mind and use that for the benefit of others.

I include the Paradoxical Commandments with the permission of Dr. Keith. In Japan too, we have a saying that the way we see the world reflects the state of our minds, and I think this coincides with Dr. Keith's poem. His Paradoxical Commandments also are in line with traditional teachings of Karma Yoga, which is what inspired me to include them here in this book. When more modern teachings, such as these Paradoxical Commandments, are conveying the same messages as traditional teachings, they can also be incorporated into tools used to assess clients' mental conditions.

The Paradoxical Commandments by Dr. Kent M. Keith

People are illogical, unreasonable, and self-centered. Love them anyway.

If you do good, people will accuse you of selfish ulterior motives. Do good anyway.

If you are successful, you will win false friends and true enemies. Succeed anyway.

The good you do today will be forgotten tomorrow. Do good anyway.

Honesty and frankness make you vulnerable. Be honest and frank anyway.

The biggest men and women with the biggest ideas can be shot down by the smallest men and women with the smallest minds. Think big anyway.

People favor underdogs but follow only top dogs. Fight for a few underdogs anyway.

What you spend years building may be destroyed overnight. Build anyway.

People really need help but may attack you if you do help them. Help people anyway.

Give the world the best you have and you'll get kicked in the teeth. Give the world the best you have anyway.

Yoga Sutras Chapter 2 Verse 36 on Truthfulness (Satya)

On being firmly established in truthfulness fruit (of action) rests on action (of the Yogi) only.

Commentary: This sutra teaches yoga practitioners the secret to living the lives they want to live, which, in other words, means living honestly and true to themselves. To live established in honesty requires being aware of one's mental state here and now, and keeping one's own thoughts, words, and deeds pure. Remember the story of the boy who

Yoga Therapy Theory

cried wolf—the boy who lied to villagers and laughed at their fear of wolves was eventually ignored when a wolf actually came. No one believed him after his numerous false alarms. This story teaches the same thing as this sutra. We must stay truthful even in times of stress so that our lives leave behind the legacy that we want. This kind of psychoeducation has been handed down in traditional yoga for thousands of years. Yoga therapists use these as standards of measure to assess clients' mental conditions, and ways of thinking and living.

Yoga Sutras Chapter 2 Verse 37 on Nonstealing (Asteya)

On being firmly established in honesty all kinds of gems present themselves (before the Yogi).

Commentary: "Honesty" in this verse is referring to that of non-misappropriativeness, or nonstealing. In our modern society, the main sources of stress are said to be human relationships, money, and pride. This sutra addresses money and the secret of how not to be controlled by how much one has. Many people think that the more money they have, the better. Traditional yoga, however, says that our wealth depends on the degree to which the desire to steal occupies our hearts. In simpler words, this sutra tells us that wealth does not stay with someone who is always greedy and full of wanting. Those who understand that they do not need what does not belong to them will find that more accumulates around them than they need. Even then, they will not claim those things as their own, will give back to society, and find that new wealth again accumulates in return. This sutra states that "all kinds of gems present themselves," but someone who does not steal in thought, word, or action, will not claim those gems as his or her own. Yoga therapists also use this verse to assess clients' mental conditions and ways of thinking and living.

Yoga Sutras Chapter 2 Verse 38 on Continence (Brahmacharya)

On being firmly established in sexual continence, vigor (is) gained.

Commentary: In traditional yoga, young ascetics did not marry and instead dedicated themselves to their discipline. This kind of discipline is called *brahmacharya*. This verse is instructing young yogis to use their life energy for their spiritual practice. This can apply to us in modern society as well, as it tells us the secret to attaining great energy. Yoga therapists can also use this verse as a reference to assess clients' mental condition.

Yoga Sutras Chapter 2 Verse 39 on Nonpossessiveness (Aparigraha)

Nonpossessiveness being confirmed there arises knowledge of the "how" and "wherefore" of existence.

Commentary: When we do not cling and are not possessive, we can see our own situations clearly. In modern, stressful, and rapidly changing societies, it is easy to lose sight of one's purpose in life. Sometimes finding meaning is difficult. Particularly in materially wealthy countries, people are not generally concerned about securing food, shelter and clothing, but many still have difficulty finding meaning. Without a clear purpose in life, there is a danger of turning to addictions, including drugs. In this sutra, we learn that if we no longer have confusion and attachment to becoming or doing something, we know precisely why we were born into this world.

This sutra contains the secret to self-realization. Yoga therapists also use this sutra as a standard to assess clients' ways of thinking and living.

Yoga Sutras Chapter 2 Verse 40 on (Physical) Cleanliness (Shaucha)

From physical purity (arises) disgust for one's own body and disinclination to come in physical contact with others.

Commentary: As I mentioned, most stress that troubles our minds can be attributed to interpersonal relationships, money, or pride. This verse is about interpersonal relationships, especially as they relate to the physical dimension. This is particularly true for young yogis, the *brahmacharis*. In industrialized countries with high divorce rates, these three stressors play havoc with our minds and disrupt our daily lives. To prevent our lives from becoming unnecessarily confused, it is best not to create complicated situations with people, money and pride. This verse teaches us it is better to simplify. Yoga therapists can also use this sutra as a standard to evaluate clients' mental conditions, ways of thinking and living.

Yoga Sutras Chapter 2 Verse 41 on (Mental) Cleanliness (Shaucha)

From mental purity (arises) purity of Sattva, *cheerful-mindedness, one-pointedness, control of the senses and fitness for the vision of the Self.*

Commentary: If we live a simplified life, then we can easily attain the one-pointedness of mind, control over the indriyas (organs in perception and action), and other qualities mentioned in this sutra. When we can live simply, focused on what is at hand, it becomes easier to accept what is happening in life and in the world around us. We know that responding to the events around us requires the clarity to see and accept them for what they are without being swayed by ideas about what other people might think. We can live as the farmer who inspired the saying, "inscrutable are the ways of heaven," and when we are ready to surrender, we become fit for the vision of the Self and are no longer swayed by the temporal world. Yoga therapists can also use this sutra as a standard to assess their clients' mental conditions and lifestyles.

Yoga Sutras Chapter 2 Verse 42 on Contentment (Santosha)

Superlative happiness from contentment.

Commentary: There is a proverb that says, "enough is as good as a feast." Contentment arises when we are able to see our own circumstances to be what is most appropriate. Maurice Maeterlinck's 1908 play, "Blue

Bird" also tells us about the importance of contentment. It is a story of a boy named Tyltyl and his younger sister Mytyl and their search for a blue bird of happiness. They are unable to find the bird until they finally return home to discover it had been there all along.

The blue bird of happiness is already in our hearts, and this is what traditional yoga teaches. It is the aim of yoga therapists to provide psychoeducation for their clients who are searching the world for the source of happiness, when it is already there within them. Yoga therapists also use this as a standard to assess their clients' mentality and lifestyle.

Yoga Sutras Chapter 2 Verse 43 on Austerities (Tapas)

Perfection of the sense organs and body after destruction of impurity by austerities.

Commentary: The austerities in this verse refer to human effort. This effort is required in any human activity like sports, art, cooking and scientific research. In yoga, it is said that those who continue tapas naturally purify their minds. This is because in order to learn and acquire knowledge and skill, you have to develop self-control. When we use the body skillfully and restrain the ten indriyas (sense organs, i.e., organs of perception and action), the mind is purified and self-control is achieved through such continued effort and discipline. For those of us living in stressful societies, self-control becomes the most powerful tool for self-protection as well. It is the job of yoga therapists to assess to what degree clients have the ability to control themselves, and then use yoga therapy techniques to build that strength.

REFERENCE 14: *PANCHADASHI* BY MAHATMA SWAMI VIDYARANYA

Chapter 1 The Differentiation of the Real Principle
Panchadashi is a sacred book written by Swami Vidyaranya Maharaji, who was the Shankara Acharya in South India Shuringeri from 1377 to 1386.

This holy place of Shuringeri is one of the four Shankara Ashrams established by the first Shankara Acharya in the seventh century. *Panchadashi* explains the teachings of Shankara Acharya in fifteen chapters, and that is why this holy book is also named *Panchadasa Prakarana* meaning "fifteen-chapter explanation." It is divided into three parts. The first part is called *Viveka Panchaka*, which explains discrimination between existence and nonexistence. The second part is called *Dipa Panchaka* and explains *Atman*, or pure consciousness of Self. The third part is called *Ananda Panchaka* in which the Bliss of Brahman is explained. In this book, it is possible to learn what Vedanta and the Upanishads are teaching. Traditional meditation techniques are also explained as follows.

Panchadashi Chapter 1 Verse 53[57]

The finding out or discovery of the true significance of the identity of the individual self and the Supreme with the aid of the great sayings (like Tattvamasi) is what is known as shravana. And to arrive at the possibility of its validity thorough logical reasoning is what is called manana.

Commentary: When using meditation to awaken to the Supreme, as explained in this verse, meditation begins with shravana (listening), and then manana, or deep deliberation and contemplation. Using the buddhi in this way to guide ourselves to realization of the real Self is not only a meditation method used to awaken to truth, it is also a useful way for yoga therapists to guide clients to more clarity in how they understand the world.

Chapter 1 Verse 54

And, when by shravana and manana the mind develops a firm and undoubted conviction, and dwells constantly on the

---

57 Vidyaranya Swami, *Panchadasi*, trans. Swami Swahananda (Chennai, India: Sri Ramakrishna Math).

thus ascertained Self alone, it is called unbroken meditation (nididhyasana).

Commentary: When one no longer has difficulty with manana, the state of nididhyasana is reached. This means that the practitioner is basically in a meditative state throughout everyday life. It is desirable that yoga therapists develop this and should ideally provide instruction to clients in this mental condition.

Chapter 1 Verse 55

When the mind gradually leaves off the ideas of the meditator and the act of meditation and is merged in the sole object of meditation (viz., the Self), and is steady like the flame of a lamp in a breezeless spot, it is called the superconscious state (samadhi).

Commentary: Charaka also taught that the state of samadhi, or moksha, a state in which the mind is free from all ignorance, is the highest state of health achievable to humankind. This verse uses the terms samadhi and moksha to mean the same thing. Many people living in our stressful societies have developed psychosomatic disorders from their daily stressors. These verses explain the importance of practicing Vedic meditation as well as abhyasa (repeated practice).

Chapter 1 Verse 62

Then the great dictum, freed from the obstacles (of doubt and ambiguity), gives rise to a direct realization of the Truth, as a fruit in one's palm—Truth that was earlier comprehended indirectly.

Yoga Therapy Theory

Commentary: Traditional yogis who overcame all the obstacles of ignorance were liberated from all worldly attachments and lived in a completely free state. Yoga therapists should also aim to guide their clients to this point. This is why yoga therapists must be able to instruct clients first in yoga therapy, and then shift into traditional yoga practices.

---

5) Prevention of Adverse Events in the Vijnanamaya Kosha

When instructing yoga therapy for the vijnanamaya kosha, yoga therapists must keep the following points in mind.

- Do not ask for more personal information than is necessary.
- Yoga therapy should begin with simple asana or pranayama. Be careful when instructing clients in meditation that involves examining past memories.
- Depending on the theme of Vedic meditation, clients might refuse to examine the topic at hand. Do not try to force them to meditate.
- Some clients might refuse to recall past events. Do not force them to do so.
- To practice meditation, it is not necessary to sit cross-legged on the floor. It is also fine to use a chair.
- Some clients will not want to admit that their way of thinking or how they use their minds is the cause of problems. Do not try to convince them of how they should think, or impose one's own value judgments by pointing out what you believe to be right and wrong in their way of thinking.
- Begin instructing clients in meditation methods that help them to have confidence (for example, remembering their accomplishments).

- The yoga therapist must maintain confidentiality in regard to any personal information about the client.
- Instruction should begin with hatha yoga practices (physical exercises), and then when the client is ready, begin meditation instruction.

6) Fictional Case Studies: Vijnanamaya Kosha

Fictional Case Study 7: Yoga Therapy for Side Effects of Hormone Therapy for Breast Cancer

1. **Introduction**

   In Japan, one in three woman gets breast cancer. But after receiving cancer treatment, many women are seeking care in facilities other than medical hospitals. In this paper, we will report the case of a woman who had severe side effects from medication and lost strength and suffered emotionally after her breast cancer operation.

2. **Client Information**

   Physical Information: Female, Age 50 years, Height 160 cm, Weight 50 kg.

   Occupation: Company employee.

   Major Complaints: Stiffness in joints and muscle pain (especially right upper arm, shoulder, and neck).

   Family Medical History: Father died from bladder cancer (age 84 years).

   Diagnosis: In January year X (age 50 years) removal of right axillary lymph node by Doctor B at Hospital A; unfavorable prognosis after surgery.

   Past Health Problems: None.

History of Current Health Problems: In January year X (age 50 years), she underwent right axillary lymph node dissection. She received radiation therapy for two months, then started hormone therapy. After five months, she started feeling pain in both shoulders and arms. Rheumatoid arthritis was suspected, but tests showed no irregularities. In September Year X, she started yoga therapy practice twice a month at her office soon after her pain started. She also began practicing at home.

Upbringing/Life Circumstances: In Year X - 7 (age 43 years), she started a small company (childcare) with her friend. Then she started a nonprofit organization, so she was essentially running a childcare business and welfare service for disabled people at the same time. She felt rewarded by her work and was constantly busy. She did not go for regular medical checkups. She went to the hospital when she started to feel unwell, and in year X - 1 (age 49 years), she happened to have a breast exam and discovered early stage breast cancer. She had an operation one month later.

Yoga Therapy History/Changes in Symptoms: In September Year X (age 50 years) she started yoga therapy twice a month for ninety minutes each time. During her intake, her main complaints were stiffness and pain in joints and muscles (right upper arm and right shoulder). We obtained her informed consent to use yoga therapy to address her complaints. Her YGPI showed mood instability. She scored depression 17/20, change of mood 12/20, sense of inferiority 11/20, sensitivity 8/20, activity 6/20, mental extroversion 11/20, and social extroversion 15/20. On the sVYASA General Health Questionnaire, her scores were 15/21 for physical health, 10/21 for emotional health, 10/21 for social health, 12/21 for spiritual health, totaling 47/84 points to put her in the "healthy" bracket. Considering these results, we began with the SSIM-YSSMA to assess her mental condition.

She scored a high 5/5 for distraction. At the beginning of her yoga therapy, we started her with easy Sukshma Vyayama. She practiced these exercises, other breathing exercises and brahmari pranayama at home every day before going to bed. In year X + 1 (age 51 years) she started to realize her own feeling of anger toward her physical condition and inability to work. We used the SSIM-AS and she scored a low 1/5 for B (ability to regulate anger). With this YTA, we found that her inability to regulate anger was one of the main causes for her major complaints. While monitoring her condition, we began counseling so that she could become more objectively aware of her body and pain. She was able to accept her situation, and then decided to seek medical treatment to address the pain. She started to take pain medication prescribed by an osteopathic clinic. Continued monitoring revealed a reduction in pain as she gained more objective awareness. She took the sVYASA General Health Questionnaire again, showing the following changes between year X and year X + 1. Physical health increase from 15 to 16/21, emotional health from 10 to 11/21, social and spiritual health did not change (from 10/21 and 12/21 respectively), making a total score change from 47 to 49/84 points. She took the test again in September X + 2 to total 70/84, and in January Year X + 3, she scored 72 points, moving her into the "very healthy" range. In Year X + 3, she started cyclic meditation and OM meditation. At this time, we assessed again using the SSIM-YSSMA, and her score improved to 1/5 for degree of distraction, and her SSIM-AS ability to regulate anger score improved to 4/5.

Client Testimony: I was lucky to join the yoga therapy class in my office, and felt much more relaxed after the first session. I was in a lot of pain at the time, so I practiced yoga therapy techniques almost every day at home, and after that the severe pain in my joints disappeared. I still take some pain medication and I feel side effects, but now I have a confidence to handle my condition by practicing yoga therapy.

3. **Observations**

    In this case study, we could clearly see that the changes in both clinical psychology tests and YTA tools were consistent. We could guide this client to become aware of her feeing of pain and anger, and we believe the changes in her attitude toward her symptoms helped her get some relief from those symptoms as well. She still has some physical difficulties, but by practicing yoga therapy techniques, she will gain the strength to cope with her physical ailments. Through continued practice, she can also develop the mental strength and continue to recover.

FICTIONAL CASE STUDY 8: YOGA THERAPY FOR EATING DISORDERS

1. **Introduction**

    Eating disorders are behavioral syndromes that have their causes in physiological and physical disorders. They often begin during adolescence when fear of weight gain begins, and the body is misunderstood to be one's true self. The main symptom is abnormal eating behaviors and is a psychological problem. Most common are anorexia nervosa and bulimia nervosa. This is a case study of a woman who suffered both disorders for fifteen years and who recovered by practicing yoga therapy.

2. **Client Information**

    Physical information: Female, Age 30 years, Height 160 cm, Weight 50 kg.

    Occupation: Housewife.

    Major Complaints: Emotional instability, anorexia, and bulimia.

    Family Medical History: None.

Diagnosis: In Year X - 10 (age 20 years), she was diagnosed by Doctor B of Hospital A with bulimia nervosa. The same year, she was diagnosed by Doctor D at Hospital G with mild depression. In year X - 7 (age 23 years), she was diagnosed by Doctor F at Hospital E with anorexia nervosa.

Past Health Problems: None.

History of Current Health Problems: In year X - 16 (age 14 years) she tried dieting after her father said she had fat legs. Her period stopped for 2 years. In Year X - 13 (age 17 years), her anorexia worsened. In year X - 2 (age 28 years), she told her husband about her anorexia after having been married five years. In Year X - 1 (age 29 years), she went to Hospital G and was diagnosed again with anorexia nervosa. She was prescribed 0.5 mmg/day of etizolam and 25 mmg/day of fluvoxamine maleate, but her symptoms became worse and she stopped taking them. The same year, her husband was hospitalized with severe headache of unknown causes. She started to study Ayurveda in hopes of being able to cure her husband. After studying Ayurveda, she started to realize that her physical condition changed and she summoned the courage to tell her classmate about her illness. After finishing the Ayurveda seminar, she joined a yoga therapy course and started to practice.

Upbringing/Life Circumstances: She was the oldest daughter in a family of four. She led an ordinary life working, getting married, and having a child, but was always unhappy about her unstable mental and physical health. At present, she lives with her husband and four-year old daughter.

Yoga Therapy History/Changes in Symptoms: She started yoga therapy in April Year X (age 30 years) and joined yoga classes seven times over a period of three months. During her intake, we first obtained her informed consent to use yoga therapy to address her complaints, then asked her to take the

Yatabe-Guilford Personality Inventory (YGPI), which showed an unhealthy mental condition. She scored 20/20 for depression, 16/20 for change of mood, 18/20 for sense of inferiority, 17/20 for sensitivity, 15/20 for lack of objectivity, and her personality type was Category E (eccentric). Her breath rate was 17 bpm, and her breathing was shallow and fast. Considering these clinical psychology tests, we used the SSIM-AS (Assessment of Spirituality). She scored a low 1/5 for ability to control attachment. To examine reasons for this, we used the SSIM-BGAK (Bhagavad Gita-based Assessment of Karma), in which she scored the lowest 1/5 for A—ability to see beyond polarity, B—ability to control the five senses, and C—ability to concentrate. Her inability in self-control was assessed to be a fundamental cause of her main complaints. We started her with breathing exercises, isometric asana breathing, and counseling using karma yoga teachings to increase her ability to control the senses. We asked her to practice every morning.

At her second session, we checked for changes in her condition, and she reported becoming more aware of her mind, and that she could eat if she tried. This indicated an improved objective understanding of her own condition, and slow training, isometric breathing exercises, sukshma vyayama, and pranayama were added to her practice.

At her third session, she seemed to be moving more actively, and she said she was once again enjoying scenery and the sensation of the wind. Considering these changes, we used the SSIM-BGAK, and she scored 4/5 for A—ability to see beyond polarity, 3/5 for B—ability to control the five senses, and 3/5 for C—ability to concentrate. Her SSIM-AS score changed from 1/5 to 4/5 for A—ability of control attachment. We added cyclic meditation and Veda meditation in May Year X to promote her range of awareness.

Her YGPI showed the following score changes in depression from 20 to 5/20, change of mood from 16 to 7/20, sense of inferiority from 18 to 6/20, sensitivity from 17 to 9/20, not-objectivity from 15 to 4/20 points and her personality type changed from E (eccentric) type to AC (average-calm) type. Her emotional instability decreased, and her activity increased. Her breath rate also changed from 17 to 12.8 times per minute. Her emotions stabilized, and we assessed she could control her anorexia and bulimia nervosa.

Client Testimony: I was suffering from my eating disorder for fifteen years and had almost given up. But after starting yoga therapy practices, I could control my symptoms and my husband's condition also improved. I feel like the fog in my brain cleared and I could control my symptoms of bulimia and anorexia. I feel more at ease in my physical body and I can now clean my house more easily. These changes feel natural, so I have confidence that I will never return to my old unhealthy condition. I hope I can keep practicing yoga therapy for a long time.

3. Observations

This client had been suffering from eating disorders for approximately 15 years. She felt superior in her ability to control herself, but inferior when things did not go the way she wanted, and the gap between these two feelings led to a lot of instability. We observed that after she could control her annamaya, pranamaya, and manomaya koshas, she could control her attachment to eating and also became more free from her anger.

Counseling and Veda meditation also helped repair her understanding in the vijnanamaya kosha and her interpretation of memories in the anandamaya kosha changed, so she could see her true worth and begin loving herself. Her husband also recovered well. We asked her to practice yoga therapy methods every morning and this healthy habit facilitated her changes. We observed that if a client has a strong will to change their bad habits, then even if the length of practice is short, the effects can be surprisingly great.

CHAPTER 5

Yoga Therapy Assessment (YTA)

and Yoga Therapy Instruction (YTI)

for the Anandamaya Kosha:

Addressing Forgotten Memories,

the Ahamkara and Chitta

1) Yoga Therapy's Pathogenesis Theory and the Anandamaya Kosha

In the anandamaya kosha in particular, ignorance from the past is stored as what I call, "forgotten memories." Forgotten memories are memories that are usually not remembered, but they contain information that creates the foundation of each individual's mentality, thus impacting behavior and the way people interpret events. Yogic practices often bring such forgotten memories to the surface, and becoming aware of them is the first step in becoming free from their influence.

The forgotten memories stored in the anandamaya kosha often influence us without our realizing it. For example, please recall the pancha kosha and human chariot theories. When information from negative memories that originate in ignorance is conveyed to the buddhi, the mistakes in cognition by the buddhi in regard to that information (such as mistaking finite for infinite, impure for pure, pain for pleasure, non-Self for Self) creates new suffering. This is because negative feelings such as attachment, bias, anxiety, and depression in regard to that information come from the buddhi.

Negative information from the buddhi in turn creates disturbances in the ten indriyas (manomaya kosha), which leads to disruption in breathing and the autonomic nervous system (pranamaya kosha), eventually causing illness in the tissues and organs of the physical body (annamaya kosha). This is how yoga therapy's pathogenesis theory is based on traditional yoga's teachings of human structure and function.

2) Yoga Therapy Assessment (YTA) and the Anandamaya Kosha

In traditional yoga philosophy, the ahamkara and chitta, two of the four psychological organs, belong to the anandamaya kosha, or the bliss sheath. The chitta functions as a storehouse of memories, and among these memories there may be trauma and other very painful memories. This negative information disrupts the decision-making and cognitive abilities of the buddhi (charioteer). Patanjali wrote in his *Yoga Sutras* that one of the goals of traditional yoga is to purify the workings of the chitta so that it is sattvic. Please see the verse that follows.

Yoga Sutras Chapter 1 Verse 2

Yoga is the inhibition of the modifications of the mind.

Commentary: I will explain more about yoga therapy techniques to "inhibit the modifications of the mind" in this chapter, but for the time being, let me say that it is necessary for yoga therapists to assess the condition of forgotten memories in the chitta (whether they are tamasic, rajasic, or sattvic). There are teachings from the *Yoga Sutras* and other scriptures that can but used as standards for assessment, and there are various tools. I will address some of these points in the following sections.

Kazuo Keishin Kimura

A. Yoga Therapy Assessment (YTA) using SOC Scale, STAI, and sVYASA General Health Questionnaire.

It is important to monitor changes from before and after practice. To do so, the initial assessment is crucial. The following references contain information useful to assess the anandamaya kosha.

REFERENCE 15: SENSE OF COHERENCE (SOC) SCALE ASSESSES THREE AREAS

Dr. Aaron Antonovsky conducted a sociological study of people who immigrated to Israel from all over the world after World War II, and after doing so, created the Sense of Coherence (SOC) scale for assessing health. People who score high on this test are said to be able to create their own health condition. According to Antonovsky's theory, this is called salutogenesis. Salutogenesis has three main factors.

1. *Comprehensibility*: the extent to which events are perceived as making logical sense, being in order, consistent, predictable and structured.
2. *Manageability*: the extent to which a person feels he/she can cope.
3. *Meaningfulness*: the extent to which a person feels that there is meaning in addressing stressful situations, or sees such situations as challenges that motivate him/her to take action.

When yoga therapists assess that a client is lacking in the preceding three factors, they can use the SOC questionnaire to gain a more detailed understanding of the client's resistance to stress. The higher the score, the higher the client's capacity to resist stress.

REFERENCE 16: ASSESSMENT OF PTSD USING IMPACT OF EVENT SCALE-REVISED VERSION (IES-R)

Yoga Therapy Theory

There are diagnostic tools used by clinical psychologists who work with people with PTSD, such as the following:

- Impact of Event Scale-Revised version (IES-R)
- Clinician Administered PTSD Scale (CAPS)

Commentary: If a client has been diagnosed with PTSD by a clinical psychologist and taken diagnostic tests, the yoga therapist should receive the client's consent to consult with the psychologist and be briefed on the results of the tests. Based on this information, the yoga therapist can then design and adjust the yoga therapy program as needed. Yoga therapists should not administer the tools themselves without having undergone the necessary education and training.

REFERENCE 17: THREE CHARACTERISTIC CATEGORIES OF PTSD SYMPTOMS

1. *Re-experiencing the traumatic event*: This may happen as "flashbacks," or in the form of dreams. If there is a situation similar to the traumatic event, then panic attacks may occur.
2. *Avoidance of reminders of trauma*: This can happen through paralysis, amnesia, dissociative identity disorder, or depersonalization disorder.
3. *Hyperarousal*: In hyperarousal, there is constant tension, insomnia, and strong irritation or anxiety.

Commentary: If yoga therapists notice any of the abovementioned symptoms, they should refer the client to a PTSD specialist and collaborate with the specialist when providing yoga therapy instruction.

B. Assess Client's Attitude toward Society

When people experience identity crises or see their identities fall apart, they may begin to harbor negative feelings toward society, such as those listed in Reference 18, and begin creating trouble in various situations. It is the job of yoga therapists to examine clients' mentality and behavior, and assess them for the forgotten memories that are at the root of disruptive behaviors.

REFERENCE 18: YTA BASED ON THE *BHAGAVAD GITA*

The following verses can be used to assess a client's attitude toward society. You may also wish to refer to the chapter on the vijnanamaya kosha for more detail on using the *Bhagavad Gita* in assessments.

Bhagavad Gita Chapter 16 Assessing Purity of Heart

Verses 1-3: *Fearlessness, purity of heart, steadfastness in Yoga and knowledge, alms-giving, control of the senses, sacrifice, study of scriptures, austerity and straightforwardness, Harmlessness, truth, absence of anger, renunciation, peacefulness, absence of crookedness, compassion toward beings, uncovetousness, gentleness, modesty, absence of fickleness, Vigor, forgiveness, fortitude, purity, absence of hatred, absence of pride—these belong to one born in a divine state, O Arjuna!*

Verse 4: *Hypocrisy, arrogance, self-conceit, harshness, and also anger and ignorance, belong to one who is born in a demoniacal state, O Arjuna!*

Verse 5: *The divine nature is deemed for liberation and the demoniacal for bondage. Grieve not, O Arjuna, for thou art born with divine properties!*

Commentary: The abovementioned teachings from the *Bhagavad Gita* are considered to be the positive and negative mental functions toward society. These mental functions and behaviors come from the buddhi (vijnanamaya kosha), but behind them are various forgotten memories residing in the chitta in the anandamaya kosha. It is necessary for yoga therapists to assess these mental functions in the process of instruction.

C. Assessing Memory Functions

In order to purify the forgotten memories in the anandamaya kosha, the client needs to try to recall them, and then use sattvic standards of intelligence (the buddhi) to correct wrong cognition. Yoga therapists assist clients in this process. A useful tool is the *Semi-Structured Manual: Assessment of Intellect and Capacity for Sensitivity and Objectivity* (SSIM-AISO) that I introduced in the previous chapter.

Yoga therapy for the anandamaya kosha is primarily instruction in meditation. In this process, clients go through past memories and do practices to purify memories themselves. Clients generally are not meditation practitioners, however, so they may have initial difficulty remembering, or may not want to remember. There are some memories that are suppressed in the chitta and are difficult to bring to the surface. It is necessary to work slowly and with care to guide the client to remember old memories and then "re-cognize" them using more healthy standards of yogic recognition. There are also cases when traumatic memories are suppressed, so the yoga therapist must be very careful, and cooperate with other professionals such as psychiatrists and psychotherapists when necessary.

D. Assess Sense of Meaning in Life

When people are unable to find meaning in life and lose a sense of purpose and identity, some begin seeking fulfillment in the senses and develop various addictions or pleasure-seeking habits. Yoga therapists need to assess clients for such tendencies. In Reference 19, I will introduce Adhi

Shankara's commentary on the *Yoga Sutras*. He wrote this commentary as one among many other scriptures some 1,300 years ago.

REFERENCE 19: ADI SHANKARA'S COMMENTARY ON THE *YOGA SUTRAS*[58]

Chapter 1 Verse 1

A clarifying illustration is given from medicine...The paralleled four-fold division of this work on yoga is as follows:
  1. *What is to be escaped (= the illness) is samsara full of pain.*

Commentary: Adi Shankara, who was born in India in the seventh century, wrote commentary on an earlier commentary of the *Yoga Sutras* by a sage named Vyasa. In Shankara's commentary, *Yoga Sutra Bhashya Vivarana*, he explains that our disease is birth into this world itself. He explains that we are born due to ignorance, and this lifetime is our chance to overcome it. If we do not take this chance, we will be born again. If we take this to heart, then yoga therapists and clients must work together, each from his/her own position, to overcome ignorance in this lifetime. Yoga therapists should do their best to help others to heal, and clients should do their best to develop self-control.

  2. *Its cause is the conjunction of Seer and seen, caused by Ignorance (avidya).*

Commentary: In this verse, Shankara Acharya says that the cause of ignorance (*avidya*) is the misrecognition of what is seen as being the Seer.

---

58 Trevor Leggett, *Sankara on the Yoga Sutras: A Full Translation of the Newly Discovered Text*. Montilal Banarsidass, Delhi, India (1992).

In yogic terms, the Seer is the true Self, the source of all life. What is seen includes everything in our world, including the five koshas which make up our bodies and minds. Shankara Acharya is basically saying that in this life, we must correct our wrong cognition that identifies ourselves with things in the temporal world. We must cure ourselves of this ignorance to liberate ourselves from this cycle of rebirth.

3. *The means of release is an unwavering (avipalva) knowledge that they are different.*

Commentary: Unless we are liberated from the temporal world, we will be continuously drawn into the changes of the world and suffer. Clients, as well as yoga therapists themselves, need to develop the wisdom and ability to discern between the Seer and the seen. Traditional yoga and yoga therapy are both among the best practices to enable this.

4. *When that Knowledge-of-the-difference (viveka-kyati) appears, Ignorance ceases: when Ignorance ceases, there is a complete end to conjunction of Seer and seen, and this is the release called kaivalya. Kaivalya (transcendental aloneness) here corresponds to the condition of health, and so it is release which is the goal*

Commentary: In this section Shankara Acharya clearly explains that those who acquire the wisdom of perfect discrimination between Seer and seen will never depend on anything in this world and will not be swayed by change. This is the Oneness in which there is no dependence, and the state that Shankara Acharya defines as perfect health. Both yoga therapy instruction and practice take the practitioner toward this goal.

REFERENCE 20: THE ASSESSMENT OF SPIRITUAL HEALTH BY DR. D. B. BISHT

Dr. D. B. Bisht, Director of Medical Education Research at the Indraprastha Apollo Hospital, New Delhi, wrote about spiritual health in his paper, "Spiritual Dimension of Health." In this paper, he mentions one way of thinking regarding characteristics of a spiritually ill person.[59] They are as follows:

a) *Greedy. Spiritually ill people are willing to take from others what does not belong to them.*
b) *Violent. Spiritually ill people are ready to hurt, maim or kill to fulfill their greed.*
c) *Afraid to lose what they have. The feeling of the need to protect is very strong. This makes giving and receiving love difficult.*
d) *Full of doubt. They have no confidence in themselves or others and cannot believe others.*
e) *Having intense desires and anger. With intense attachments, people lose perception of themselves.*

Commentary: As Dr. Bisht says, it is easy to assess whether someone is liberated or not by examining the degree of harmony in their relations with others and the world around them. Yoga therapists can use the above as standards to assess the spiritual health of the client. At JYTS, we have created the *Semi-Structured Interview Manual: Assessment of Spirituality* (SSIM-AS) that yoga therapists can use as a reference when asking questions to the client and observing the client's behavior.

———

E. Ayurveda-Based Assessment

Charaka explained the final goal of medical treatment as guiding the patient to moksha, or liberation. Though liberation is not generally thought of as in the realm of medical science, there are some important points

---

59 Bisht, "Spiritual Dimensions of Health," 125.

worth considering from the perspectives of medicine and clinical psychology. I will introduce some of them in Reference 21.

––––––

REFERENCE 21: THE FINAL GOAL OF TREATMENT

Charaka Samhita: Sharira Sthana Chapter I Verses 94–97

Absolute eradication of miseries is obtained by the elimination of desires. Desire is the root cause of all miseries. Elimination of desires lends to the eradication of all miseries. A silkworm provides for itself suicidal threads. So does an ignorant person, bound with worldly miseries, provides for himself desires arising out of the various objects. A wise person, who abstains from the objects of senses, considering them as dangerous as burning fire does not subject himself to any wishful acts and contacts with their objects with the result that miseries never overcome him.

Commentary: It is as if Charaka were writing for people today who are suffering from modern lifestyle diseases. We all know how easy it is to become fond of things that are not good for our health, and when that tendency goes too far, it can lead to psychosomatic disorders. This is what Charaka is explaining in this verse.

So, why are clients unable to resist the temptations of things that are not good for them? It is due to the temptations that arise from the forgotten memories, the samskara, that reside in the chitta in the anandamaya kosha. Clients do not yet possess sufficiently sharp and strong intellect and sensitivity to overcome the temptations of the sense organs. Speaking in yoga therapy terms, the problem lies with ignorance in the buddhi, the psychological organ that holds the reins of the indriya, the 10 organs of perception and action. Traditional Raja Yoga is one method to strengthen the function of the buddhi, so yoga therapists should provide psychoeducation to their clients through Raja Yoga practice to cultivate the functioning of the buddhi.

Charaka Samhita: Sharira Sthana Chapter I Verse 99

If something eternal is viewed as ephemeral, and something harmful as useful and vice versa, this is indicative of the impairment of intellect. For the Intellect normally views things as they are.

Commentary: As I explained in the chapter on the vijnanamaya kosha, when there is ignorance, things are not seen for what they are, and wrong cognition occurs. The client's wrong cognition needs to be assessed, and by imparting traditional yogic teachings and providing instruction in yoga therapy techniques as psychoeducation, the yoga therapist can guide the client to better health.

Charaka Samhita: Sharira Sthana Chapter I Verses 130–131

Neither the sense organs nor their objects alone can bring about happiness or miseries. The latter are in fact caused by the four-fold combination mentioned above (viz., proper utilization, wrong utilization, excessive utilization, and non-utilization). Even if there are sense organs and their objects present, there would be no disease, nor any happiness unless the four-fold combination is involved. So this combination itself constitutes a causative factor for happiness and miseries.

Commentary: Before this verse, Charaka explains that disease is caused by the wrong, excessive, or inadequate use of the senses (*Charaka Samhita* 4.1.127–128). In addition to these three uses, there is proper utilization of the senses, making uses of the sense organs fourfold. In this verse, Charaka is saying that happiness and misery depend on the way we use the senses—they can be used properly, improperly, excessively, or not at all.

The sense organs usually function to collect information from outside of ourselves. The ten horses are always looking outward, but to interrupt that tendency and bring our attention inward can correct or alleviate the excessive outward-going tendencies that bring about psychosomatic illnesses. Yoga therapists use modified traditional yoga techniques to guide the clients in doing so.

Charaka Samhita: Sharira Sthana Chapter I Verses 138–139

Happiness and miseries are felt due the contact of the Soul, the sense organs, mind and the objects of senses. Both these types of sensations disappear when the mind is concentrated and contained in the Soul and the super-natural powers in the mind and body are attained. This state is known as yoga according to sages well versed in this science.

Commentary: In these verses, Charaka refers to yoga. He defines the state of yoga as being when the functions of pure consciousness from the life principle/Self are able to keep the inner psychological organs from going outward to connect with external objects. In other words, the mind is steadily concentrated on the Self. Vyasa also says the same in his fifth-century commentary on the *Yoga Sutras*. Vyasa uses "yoga" to mean "samadhi," the highest state of concentration. "But the concentration attained by a mind which is one-pointed, i.e. occupied with one thought, which brings enlightenment about a real entity, weakens the kleshas, loosens the bonds of Karma and paves the way to the arrested state of the mind, is called Samprajnata yoga."[60]

---

60 Swami Hariharananda Aranya, *Yoga Philosophy of Patanjali: Containing His Yoga Aphorisms with Vyasa's Commentary in Sanskrit and a Translation with Annotations Including Many Suggestions for Practice of Yoga*, 1st edition, translated by P. N. Mukherji (New York: State University of New York Press, 1984), 2.

In the scriptures, yoga and samadhi are sometimes used as synonyms, when they refer to being in the highest state completely unhindered by the matters of the world. This state of consciousness is the key to our transcendence of happiness and misery, and it is one of the central tenents guiding yoga therapy instruction.

Charaka Samhita: Sharira Sthana Chapter I Verse 142

Moksha or salvation is nothing but an absolute detachment of all contacts by virtue of the absence of rajas and tamas in the mind and annihilation of effects of potent past actions. This is a state after which there are no more physical or mental contacts.

Commentary: In order to guide a client to perfect health, the yoga therapist must help the client bring the sattvic state of mind into predominance. But even in that state, rajas and tamas will not cease to exist. While explaining the traditional philosophy of yoga, Charaka says that if one is able to maintain a sattvic state of mind to overcome each moment with a steady mind, it will lead to conquering all past lives and past events. Traditional yoga teaches us that liberation from the past depends on how we act in the present. Indian yogis believe that if one is able to do this, then there is no more need to be reborn into this world of suffering.

Charaka Samhita: Sharira Sthana Chapter I Verses 143–146

The following serve as means to the attainment of moksha.
  1. Due devotion to noble Souls
  2. Shunning of the company of the wicked
  3. Observing sacred vows and fasts
  4. Pursuit of the rules of good conduct
  5. Compliance with scriptural prescriptions
  6. Scriptural knowledge

Yoga Therapy Theory

7. Liking for lonely living
8. Detachment from the objects of senses
9. Striving for moksha (salvation)
10. Absolute mental control
11. Abstinence from the performance of acts leading to good and sinful effects
12. Annihilation of the effects of past-actions
13. Desire to get away from the worldly trap
14. Absence of egoistic disposition
15. Being afraid of contacts of the Soul, the mind, and the body
16. Concentration of the mind and intellect in the Soul; and
17. Review of spiritual facts

All this can be attained by virtue of the constant remembering of the fact that the Soul is different from the body and the latter has nothing to do with the former.

Commentary: In this verse, Charaka explains how to draw out our capacity to awaken to Reality, the tendency that guides us to the state of emancipation. This would be no surprise coming from a master of yoga, but Charaka was a physician. For Charaka to be able to explain ways to complete one's spiritual journey proves that Ayurveda is the mind-body medicine of life that guides clients to a perfect state of mind. Yoga therapists should also try to live with this state of mind and guide clients toward the same.

Charaka Samhita: Sharira Sthana Chapter I Verses 150–151

The power of metaphysical memory constitutes the best way of liberation, as shown by the liberated ones. Persons following this way do not come back to worldly traps. This is again the best way to the attainment of yoga (communion with God) as well as moksha (salvation). This is what the yogins, the virtuous ones, the followers of the Sankhya system, and the liberated ones say.

Commentary: Charaka says that the state of ultimate health is the emancipated state of mind. This is the aim of yoga, and yoga therapists should strive to achieve this state of mind with their clients. For this purpose, yoga therapists and their clients should not limit their goal to eliminating symptoms, but should begin the practice of traditional yoga after symptoms are relieved, to aim for the highest emancipated state of mind.

Charaka Samhita: Sharira Sthana Chapter I Verses 152–153

Anything that has a cause constitutes misery; it is alien and ephemeral. It is not produced by the Soul (Atman); but one has got a feeling of its ownership until one has got a real knowledge to the effect that this is something different from him; and is not his own. As soon as one knows it, he gets rid of all (miseries).

Commentary: We mistake the five koshas of the pancha kosha theory to be who we are, ourselves. This is the reason for our misery, as all of the koshas have a cause and are ephemeral. The mental practice of observing these thoughts and quieting them is called *samyama* in traditional yoga, and this is practiced by yogis. This practice is important to do for both yoga therapists and clients.

Charaka Samhita: Sharira Sthana Chapter I Verse 154

As soon as the final renunciation in respect of all subsequent actions is attained, the very consciousness together with its final causes in the form of indeterminate, determinate, or scriptural knowledge is completely eradicated.

Commentary: Charaka is explaining that the ultimate state is when "the very consciousness together with its final causes" is "completely

Yoga Therapy Theory

eradicated." Charaka is saying precisely the same thing that is brought to light in yoga philosophy. It is indeed possible that Charaka himself was a yogi.

———

In Reference 21, I commented on Charaka's exposition of the perfect state of human health. Yoga therapists also use Ayurvedic assessments to guide their clients to the ultimate state of health. This concludes a cursory explanation of yoga therapy assessment for the *anandamaya kosha*.

3) PRINCIPLES OF YOGA THERAPY INSTRUCTION (YTI) FOR THE ANANDAMAYA KOSHA

Traditional yoga teaches us that the key to finding our primordial existence is self-control. Self-control in and of itself is liberation from the temporal world. Swami Krishnananda of the Sivananda Ashram Divine Life Society said, "self-control is also Self-realization."[61]

4) PURIFICATION OF AND INSTRUCTION FOR THE ANANDAMAYA KOSHA

The main means to purify the anandamaya kosha, the innermost kosha, is meditation. There are two main kinds of meditation for this purpose, namely Veda meditation and Raja Yoga meditation. Veda meditation involves listening to an explanation of the theme of meditation (shravana), then considering it intently (manana) (see reference 14). Raja Yoga meditation for ordinary people is bringing attention to your breath coming in and out of the body, or to the heartbeat (see reference 23 Verse 34).

Psychoeducation as done in the four major paths of yoga, is very important for the anandamaya kosha. Yoga therapists should, therefore, teach the philosophy of Jnana Yoga, Bhakti Yoga, Karma Yoga, and Raja Yoga

---

61 Swami Krishnananda, *Epistemology of Yoga*, 186 (e-book edition).

to clients, and while assessing the clients' values, guide them to become aware of the flaws in their beliefs that lead to disease. Then yoga therapists can guide clients with meditation to become objectively aware of their forgotten memories and remedy the mistaken cognition of those memories.

In this way, clients can gradually acquire both mental and physical self-control. It is by working on the *anandamaya kosha* that one strives to achieve not only physical, mental and social health, but also spiritual health, or ultimately the perfect state of health.

Next, I will introduce verses from the *Brihadaranyaka Upanishad* about Veda meditation.

———

REFERENCE 22: *BRIHADARANYAKA UPANISHAD* VOLUME 4 CHAPTER 5 VERSE 6

The dialog between Yajnavalkya and his wife (teachings on Vedic Meditation)

This Self has to be realized. Hear about this Self and meditate upon him, Maitreyi. When you hear about the Self, meditate upon the Self, and finally realize the Self, you come to understand everything in life.

Commentary: Vedic meditation is introduced in the *Brihadaranyaka Upanishad*, which makes up a significant portion of the *Upanishads*, written four to five thousand years ago. Vedic meditation has four steps, namely, (1) shravana (listening), (2) manana (contemplation), (3) nididhyasana (meditation in daily life), and (4) jnana (realization). Yogis from ancient times practiced these four steps of meditation to realize Truth.

I too practiced this way when I studied with my guru Swami Yogeshwarananda Maharaji in the Himalayas. My guru would speak to us for about one hour before meditation, and we would listen intently (shravana). Then every morning and evening, he would instruct us in meditation in such a way that we could contemplate deeply about the topic he gave us

Yoga Therapy Theory

(manana). We did this twice a day, every day, and in addition, when we were at the ashram, we would continue contemplating in our daily life (nididhyasana). In this way, we attained realization (jnana) of many gems of wisdom. Yoga therapists can adapt teachings from traditional Vedic meditation to suit the mental condition of the client, to guide the client to deeper insight.

REFERENCE 23: PATANJALI'S *YOGA SUTRAS* ON RAJA YOGA MEDITATION

In Patanjali's *Yoga Sutras*, Raja Yoga meditation methods are introduced to purify the chitta. I will explain some of them that follow. It will be evident to you how traditional yoga is a practice that purifies through to the depths of the human psyche.

Chapter 1 Verse 2

Yoga is the inhibition of the modifications of the mind.

Commentary: "Mind" in this verse is chitta. This verse is thereby implying that yoga is a method to purify the psyche, all the way to forgotten memories stored in the chitta. Concrete techniques are introduced in the *Yoga Sutras* from verse 33, and I will include some of them here. The techniques are impossible to convey only with words, so for actual instruction, I recommend receiving instruction from a qualified yoga psychotherapist who understands these principles.

Chapter 1 Verse 33

The mind becomes clarified by cultivating attitudes of friendliness, compassion, gladness and indifference respectively toward happiness, misery, virtue and vice.

Commentary: Patanjali's *Yoga Sutras* are well known as the authoritative text of Raja yoga. "Raja" means "king," and Raja Yoga is known as such the "King of Yoga" because it includes techniques from all other categories

225

of yoga. This verse introduces a Karma yoga purification method. When we see people who are happy, we should celebrate their happiness in a way that the happiness increases, and when someone is suffering, we should have compassion for that person. When someone does something good, we should share in their joy and try to forget their bad deeds, even if we were the ones who suffered from them. Through such daily karma, good memories will accumulate in people who live this way. This is why attitudes in daily life and daily habits are important in both traditional yoga and in yoga therapy.

Chapter 1 Verse 34

Or by the expiration and retention of breath.

Commentary: This verse is a continuation from the previous one, providing another method for mental purification. It is clear from this verse that pranayama, the fourth limb of yoga, is also related to purification of memories. Therapists from JYTS are working with clients who are struggling with their past and PTSD, as well as with people who have extreme anxiety and who are suffering from agoraphobia. In both cases, we are seeing beneficial effects of yoga therapy, and one of the methods we use is pranayama. It is impossible to do pranayama without bringing your attention to the here and now, because you must be present to be aware of your breath. This is part of the mechanism of how pranayama is helpful for people with trauma or anxiety, and it is beneficial as mental training. Such training helps to purify even anxious minds.

Chapter 1 Verse 37

Also the mind fixed on those who are free from attachment (acquires steadiness).

Commentary: Those who are free from attachment are good role models for how to live. When we try to imitate and adopt such mentality, we

Yoga Therapy Theory

also develop the same detachment from worldly affairs, and purify the *chitta*. Such psychological techniques are used in both traditional yoga and in yoga therapy.

Chapter 1 Verse 38

Also (the mind) depending upon the knowledge derived from dreams or dreamless sleep (will acquire steadiness).

Commentary: In traditional yoga theory, the four stages of mind are (1) waking state, (2) dream state, (3) sound sleep state, and (4) the forth state (*turiya*). In our daily lives, we observe the dream and sleep states. We know that we have dreamed, or we know that we slept soundly, or we sometimes know that we are dreaming. This means that deep within us, there is a presence that is constantly aware of our mental functions, whether we are awake or asleep. In traditional yoga, this deep inner consciousness is used to distance ourselves from worldly affairs and passions to achieve a liberated state of mind. For this purpose, traditional yoga practices have been transmitted over thousands of years. Among them is the teaching in the next verse.

Chapter 1 Verse 39

Or by meditation as desired.

Commentary: Meditation is not about just sitting without thinking. While it is important to develop the ability to become absorbed in meditation, there are other things that a beginning practitioner must do first to calm the mind. I too spent years studying many techniques under my guru, Swami Yogeshwarananda Maharaj. My guru assessed the mental condition of his students, and then chose the meditation technique appropriate for each individual. In yoga therapy as well, therapists must select the best meditation method for the client after assessing the client's mental condition. Instruction in appropriate meditation techniques will help to purify forgotten memories. This kind of psychotherapy is very sensitive work, however, so it is important to follow the instructions of a certified yoga therapist.

———

Chapter 2 of the *Yoga Sutras* explains the mechanism by which meditation is effective. I will introduce some of the verses that follow.

———

REFERENCE 24: PATANJALI'S *YOGA SUTRAS* CHAPTER 2

Chapter 2 Verse 10

These, the subtle ones, can be reduced by resolving them backward into their origin.

Commentary: This verse is talking about klesha-s, or "afflictions," which are (1) ignorance, (2) sense of self ("I-am-ness"), (3) attraction toward objects, (4) repulsion, and (5) strong desire for life. In the *Yoga Sutras*, Patanjali says that these afflictions can be overcome if attention is turned to their causes and the causes understood. This is what is meant by reducing *kleshas* by "resolving them backward into their origin." This is a traditional yoga technique, similar to modern day cognitive therapy. The mental function that is at the foundation of the affliction is brought into awareness and re-examined. With re-examination, cognition changes and affliction is overcome. This has been taught in traditional yoga for thousands of years. It is clear that a critical part of yoga therapy is finding the causes of unhealthy mental functions, and then changing cognition to one that is psychologically healthy.

Chapter 2 Verse 11

Their active modifications are to be suppressed by meditation.

Yoga Therapy Theory

Commentary: In this section, meditation is mentioned as a way to overcome unhealthy mental functions. Afflictions can be eliminated with meditative psychotherapy. This is because dhyana (meditation) is a traditional practice in which you can sit quietly, forget about your body and breathing, and turn your attention solely to your psychological functions. Through this Vedic meditation, one after another, forgotten memories are seen in a different light. This new and clearer cognition of past events lessens internal conflict and suffering. This is a traditional yoga practice and is now a modern yoga psychotherapy technique.

Chapter 2 Verse 12

The reservoir of Karmas that are rooted in Kleshas brings all kinds of experiences in the present and future lives.

Commentary: The chitta, which is the storehouse of old memories, belongs to the innermost anandamaya kosha. The various unhealthy memories which are sources of afflictions are also in this kosha. The "reservoir of Karmas" can be thought of as impressions left by previous actions. These impressions in turn influence an individual's actions and psychological functions. As long as unhealthy motivators are active, they will lead a person to unhealthy behavior. This results in manifestation "in the present and future lives." This is why yoga therapists provide instruction that helps clients recall unhealthy memories in the chitta and become aware of their unhealthy cognition, and then guide them to healthy cognition and liberation from a life of ignorance.

Chapter 2 Verse 16

The misery which is not yet come can and is to be avoided.

Commentary: If old memories that create unhealthy motivations can be seen from a healthy perspective, ignorance can be eliminated and future suffering can also be prevented. Traditional meditation techniques can be used in modern yoga therapy. However, yoga therapists must exercise caution when encouraging clients to go inward, as unexpected suppressed memories may arise. These practices are not to be done frivolously. The practitioner must be ready not only to recall the past, but also have the tools to objectively and calmly observe memories, no matter how painful they may be. For this purpose, yoga therapy begins with yoga therapy breathing exercises that help clients become aware of their physical dimension. Clients thus develop the ability to observe first their body and then the breath. After helping the client develop the necessary awareness and strength, yoga therapists can instruct clients in meditation practices such as the Vedic meditation and Raja yoga meditation mentioned in this book.

Chapter 2 Verse 17

The cause of that which is to be avoided is the union of the Seer and the Seen.

Commentary: This verse contains the two concepts of Seer and the seen. These were also introduced in the chapter on the vijnanamaya kosha, so you may wish to refer back to the previous chapter. This verse tells us that all causes of suffering are removed when we can observe all things objectively and no longer identify with the temporal, including the five koshas. Afflictions emerge due to the inability to be objective, and even though traditional practices are ancient, they can help people in modern societies to become aware of the roots of their psychological functions. This enables new meaning and insight to arise. This is what modern yoga therapy instruction is about.

Chapter 2 Verse 23

The purpose of the coming together of the Purusha *and* Prakrti *is gaining by the* Purusha *of the awareness of its true nature and the unfoldment of powers inherent in Purusha and Prakrti.*

Yoga Therapy Theory

Commentary: Many questions challenge us. Why do Purusha and Prakrti exist separately? Why are some people saintly and others devilish? Why is there the eternal and temporal? Why are the body and mind constantly changing? This verse explains the reason as being for "the unfoldment of powers inherent in Purusha and Prakrti." Because some people are evil, others strive to be good; because we are surrounded by what is limited, we search for that which is eternal; because the body and mind are ever changing, we strive to become an immoveable presence. The scriptures tell us that these efforts enable our inner divine power to unfold. Because we, as yoga practitioners, also find ourselves suffering due to our attachment to the changing world, we practice traditional yoga and yoga therapy in the hope of transcending that changing world. This is also an "unfolding of inherent powers." Yoga therapists can light the fire of earnestness in the client, and work to help clients discover their own ability to free themselves from suffering.

Chapter 2 Verse 24

Its cause is the lack of awareness of one's Real nature.

Commentary: Though our modern society is generally said to be stressful, not everyone suffers from stress-related disorders. Disorders arise when clients lose themselves in the "coming together of Seer and seen." For example, people with addictions develop strong connections with the "seen" (object of addiction) and identify with the addiction as their own nature to the degree that they cannot detach from it. This mental condition is avidya, translated in this verse as "lack of awareness" and also often translated as "ignorance." Avidya—ignorance of our true nature—is the beginning of suffering, and most people in our modern societies have this to varying degrees. It is important that each of us develops the ability to discriminate between "that which I observe" and "the I who is observing." It is the job of the yoga therapist to teach the techniques that enable awareness of and the ability to differentiate between the two to be developed.

Chapter 2 Verse 25

The dissociation of Purusha and Prakrti brought about by the dispersion of Avidya is the real remedy and that is the Liberation of the Seer.

Commentary: In Sanskrit, the word for health is *swasth*—"swa" meaning self, and *"asth"* meaning existence. The concept of health in Sanskrit involves an individual's ability to "exist by oneself" without being dependent on anyone. Realization of the true Self frees a person from any dependence. There is a hypothesis that this word for health traveled from India to the West, where the sound "swa" became "ha" in the Middle East, and eventually *"swasth"* became "health."[62] If this is correct, the origin of the English word "health" shares the meaning with the Sanskrit compound, "to stay in the Self." This is the "dispersion of Avidya," the "real remedy," the "Liberation of the Seer." There is no dependence on anything else. To stay in the Self is the ultimate state of health.

Chapter 2 Verse 26

The uninterrupted practice of the awareness of the Real is the means of dispersion (of Avidya).

Commentary: To achieve the ultimate state of health described in Verse 25, we must make constant effort to be aware of the real Self, and to identify ourselves with that. When yoga therapists provide instruction to clients, they guide clients to acquire wisdom and the discriminative ability to differentiate between the Seer and the seen. For example, misidentification of oneself with one's profession is a common source of stress.

---

62 Bisht, "Spiritual Dimensions of Health," 122.

When a person's identity is tied to their job, losing the job could create an identity crisis and tremendous stress. With clarity and the ability to see the difference between one's Self and one's occupation, the stress of losing one's job is significantly reduced.

---

5) PREVENTION OF ADVERSE EVENTS IN THE ANANDAMAYA KOSHA

I have explained the basic theories of yoga therapy and yoga therapy assessment based on Raja Yoga scriptures and the *Yoga Sutras.* In this section, I list some points of caution for yoga therapists engaged in this kind of yoga therapy. For yoga instructors who are interested in contributing to society by providing instruction to people suffering from stress-related illnesses and struggling with fundamental identity issues, I would encourage you to study yoga therapy from the basics and empower yourself with the knowledge that traditional yoga and the scriptures impart.

- Yoga therapists should not ask clients for unnecessary personal information.
- Yoga Therapy should start with simple asana and breathing exercises. Meditation should be introduced carefully when the client is ready.
- If clients do not follow instructions or resist meditation instructions, yoga therapists should not insist upon doing meditation.
- Some clients may resist or refuse to look into the content of the anandamaya kosha (i.e., painful memories). Yoga therapists must not pressure clients to do so.
- If clients have difficulty sitting on the floor, meditation can also be done sitting in a chair.
- Meditation instruction should be divided into beginner, intermediate, and advanced practices. It is best to begin Vedic meditation with positive themes that are easier to reflect upon.

6) Fictional Case Studies: Anandamaya Kosha

Fictional Case Study 9: Yoga Therapy for Anxiety due to Excessive Drinking

1. **Introduction:**

Memories from infancy can affect a person over a lifetime. When these forgotten memories involve neglect or self-negation, it becomes particularly difficult to maintain a positive self-image, even as adults. This client suffered from self-negation that she developed growing up, from when she was a child into her life as a working adult. She read a book about trauma and yoga and decided to seek help through yoga therapy. This is a clinical report of her case.

2. **Client Information:**

Physical Information: Female, Age 35 years, Height 152 cm, Weight 48 kg.

Occupation: Company Employee.

Major Complaints: Excessive intake of alcohol, self-consciousness, sudden fear, fatigue.

Family Medical History: Father died from stomach cancer (age 73 years). Mother has high blood pressure (age 70 years), coronary artery stenosis.

Diagnosis: none.

Past Health Problems: Autonomic Imbalance (age 24 years), Insomnia and took etizolam tablets 0.4 mg/day for one year (age 30 years).

History of current health problems: Year X - 23 (age 12 years), she was ignored by friends at primary school. She was unable to tell anyone about her problems and began wishing she would disappear. In year X - 21 (age 14 years) her family moved to another region, and she made new friends but always worried they would betray her. In year X - 15 (age 20 years), she started working at an office and tried to be positive and cheerful with new friends. But she still was afraid her friends would call her names and she began inflicting self-injury by cutting her abdomen. In Year X - 7 (age 28 years) she divorced and returned to her hometown. She had severe stress raising her child and living with her parents again. She also had financial difficulties and worried about her future. She sometimes felt she might lose mental balance. Every day she felt fatigue, general malaise, and self-reproach. She sometimes would drink alcohol and take out her anger on her family. Year X (age 35 years) she read the book, *Overcoming Trauma Through Yoga* and found that one client's life in the book was quite similar to hers, so she started attending yoga classes.

Upbringing/Life Circumstances: Her father was a bank employee, and her mother worked in the service industry. Her father sometimes came home drunk and would verbally and physically abuse her mother, so she always felt uneasy when her father was at home. She was one of two children, and as a child, she had a bright and active personality, but got angry when she did not get her own way. After graduating from a technical college, she got a job and moved to another prefecture. She became pregnant soon after, had a baby, and got married. Later she divorced and returned home. She now lives with her mother and child and also has a job.

Yoga Therapy History/Changes in Symptoms: In August year X (age 35 years) she started yoga therapy once a week at her yoga therapist's home. She told the yoga therapist about her tendency to drink. At her first yoga therapy session, the therapist first obtained her informed consent to use yoga therapy to address her complaints. Then she took the YGPI, which indicated her mentally unhealthy condition. She scored depression 15/20, change of mood 11/20, sense of inferiority 9/20, sensitivity 8/20. She also scored activeness 7/20, outward thinking 9/20, outward activity 10/20. Her emotional instability was evident in her scores. Her STAI trait anxiety score was 44, and state anxiety 42, indicating strong tendencies for anxiety. Considering her initial test results, SSIM-BGAK (Bhagavad Gita-based Assessment of Karma) was used to assess her ability to control her senses. She scored 2/5 for ability to control sense organs. To strengthen self-control, her program began with isometric breathing exercises. In September of the same year, it was evident that she would become tense when speaking with other people. The therapist assessed that she was tense due to excessive concern about being seen by people around her. The following month she noticed a decrease in tension. We used the SSIM-AS (Assessment of Spirituality) to assess her anandamaya kosha as she spoke about being ignored by others, and she scored a low 2/5 for ability to control doubt toward others. We assessed that this was one the main causes of her complaints and began Vedic meditation the same month. She was asked to remember times when she was successful, and that helped her to speak in more positive terms about herself. She began opening up and cried while showing the yoga therapist the scars on her abdomen. After four months of yoga therapy practice, she also began to notice her own tension and started to regulate her own mental and physical balance utilizing breathing techniques. During this same period, the therapist also assessed that her sudden onsets of fear and heaviness in her head were among the three symptoms of PTSD. Sukshma vyayama, isometric breathing, and isometric sukshma vyayama were added to her program. This helped bring her attention inward, in particular to the way she was using her body. After six months of yoga therapy, she became aware of when she would start dissociating and was able to objectively notice her own condition. She noticed that if she heard someone speak angrily or witnessed violence, she would feel very heavy in her head and felt fear of not being able to escape. She was able to reduce her alcohol intake, and her SSIM-BGAK score for ability to control the senses increased to 4/5.

Her ability to see her condition objectively continued to improve over the year, and she gained better control of her senses. She became aware that her instability had its roots in trauma as an infant. She said she wanted to stop living an unhealthy lifestyle and wanted to choose to be happy. At this point, she took the YG test again. Her marks showed improvement. Her depression score improved from 15 to 10/20, change of mood from 11 to 7/20, sense of inferiority from 9 to 4/20, and sensitivity from 8 to 4/20. Her activeness score improved from 7 to 10/20, outward thinking from 9 to 12/20, and outward activity from 10 to 15/20. Her STAI scores improves, trait anxiety going from 44 to 34, and state anxiety 42 to 31. Her SSIM-AS regulation of doubt improved from 2 to 4/5.

Client Testimony: My emotional instability as a child continued into adulthood, and sometimes I took things out on people around me. No matter who I was with, I always felt alone and anxious, but when I did yoga, I felt happiness and a feeling of warmth. I practiced pranayama and isometric breathing exercises using my hands, and I could feel my symptoms getting better, and I overcame my anxiety about having fear. I can observe myself better now, and I realized that the source of my suffering has always been the same. I realized I was carrying baggage and that I could put it down and choose to be happy. I stopped checking to see what other people were thinking of me, and slowly, I have become able to live my own life. I never told people about my past, but after I told the yoga therapist and cried, I felt much better. I want to be able to face my past now.

3. **Observations**

Everyone is affected by the cumulative influences of the past, but in this client's case, by practicing yoga therapy that enabled her to overcome her self-negating tendencies, she could see her past experiences in a different light. This is the power of self-healing that yoga therapy enables. She cured herself of her own excessive drinking and other unhealthy habits and started living a healthier life. The improvement in her symptoms was evident in her changing scores in both clinical psychology as well as yoga therapy's SSIMs. Yoga therapy has great potential as a psychotherapy to overcome trauma.

FICTIONAL CASE STUDY 10: YOGA THERAPY FOR PTSD FROM EARTHQUAKE DISASTER

1. Introduction

A woman who experienced the Great East Japan earthquake had difficulty being in crowded places and could not relax in the living room of her residence, which had been damaged by the earthquake. She felt safest in bed in her second-floor bedroom. She felt stiffness in her shoulders and heaviness in her body and had no motivation to move. She suspected that these symptoms were due to trauma from the earthquake and decided to try yoga therapy as a way to overcome it. In this paper, we consider the validity of yoga therapy to change the relationship between body and mind.

2. Client Information

Physical Information: Female, Age 55 years, Height 160 cm, Weight 50 kg.

Occupation: Office Worker.

Major Complaints: Heaviness, still shoulders, constipation, edema, anxiety, irritation.

Family Medical History: Father (age 92 years) and mother (age 87 years) high blood pressure; second son (age 28) brain infarction (age 15 years) and recurrence (ages 18 and 23 years), atopic dermatitis, nasal allergy.

Diagnosis: None.

Yoga Therapy Theory

Past Health Problems: Year X - 43 (age 12 years) and year X - 23 (age 32 years) Autonomic imbalance diagnosed at Hospital A. Year X - 9 (age 46 years) carpal tunnel syndrome diagnosed at Hospital B. Year X - 6 (age 49 years) asthma/supraventricular tachycardia diagnosed at Hospital C.

History of Current Health Problems: In Year X - 1 (age 54 years), she experienced the Great East Japan Earthquake. Her house was partially destroyed. She was without electricity and water supply for ten days and had no gas supply for one month. She could not go to work by subway for two months and had to use the bus instead. Her workload increased after the earthquake, and she felt a lot of stress. After lifelines were restored and her house was repaired, life basically returned to pre-earthquake conditions. During a New Year gathering at her office, she felt so much constriction in her chest and difficulty breathing when she tried to enter a room full of people that she had to leave.

At about that time, she also felt uncomfortable in her living room and felt calmest when in bed. She developed a strong dislike for crowded buses and subways, so she started leaving her house early to avoid rush hour. She put on weight and developed edema, constipation, stiff shoulders, and a dislike for exercise. She suspected that this was due to trauma from the earthquake, and in year X (age 55 years), she started yoga therapy.

Upbringing/Life Circumstances: She was shy from a young age and was not good at being with people. She tended to care too much about what others were thinking. In year X - 23 (age 32 years), she became dizzy when standing up and developed anxiety and felt pressure in her chest. She was diagnosed with autonomic imbalance and rested for three months at home. In year X - 9 (age 46 years) she was diagnosed with carpal tunnel syndrome. Around that time, her office announced restructuring, and she felt very anxious. In year X - 7 (age 48 years) she was diagnosed with asthma and supraventricular tachycardia at

Hospital C. She began feeling it too bothersome to meet people, felt a lot of tension, and lost confidence in her ability to regulate her own condition. In year X - 6 (age 49 years) she began participating in yoga therapy classes.

Yoga Therapy History/Changes in Symptoms: After the earthquake, she was unable to do yoga for about a year, but she started doing breathing exercises before work. In year X (age 55 years), she resumed yoga therapy and after giving informed consent to use yoga therapy to address her complaints, she started an anti-ageing yoga therapy program and yoga therapy asana to recover muscle strength. Her POMS T value was tension-anxiety 76, depression 78, anger-hostility 75, vigor 53, fatigue 74, and confusion 76. Considering the POMS results and her irritability when practicing the anti-ageing yoga therapy program, we used the SSIM-YSSMA (Yoga Sutra-based State of Mind Assessment). We found that her inability to attain higher levels (lack of goals) marked a high 5/5, and this was one of the reasons for her main complaints. We decided to first instruct her in pranayama at her own pace, but her breath was shallow and fast, and she could not breathe from her diaphragm. Since disturbance in her pranamaya kosha was most pronounced, we persisted in her pranayama instruction, and after some time she was able to breathe deeply and consciously. By two years after the earthquake, she had a regular home practice; her heaviness, shoulder stiffness, and back pain had all been eased, and her constipation and edema improved. She spoke happily of how light she felt, and her SSIM-YSSMA inability to attain higher levels (lack of goals) improved from 5/5 to 2/5. The T value of her POMS also improved: tension-anxiety from 76 to 70, depression from 78 to 72, anger-hostility from 75 to 70, vigor from 53 to 59, fatigue from 74 to 70, confusion from 76 to 70. While this showed improvement as a whole, the scores indicate she is still strongly influenced by unhealthy emotions and that the trauma is still strongly rooted.

Client Testimony: During the earthquake, the ground in my garden cracked open, and my house tilted over. Damage was greatest in the living room, where the glass door came off, the window glass broke, and all the things in the room were scattered everywhere. My house sank ten centimeters into the ground, especially in the living room. We repaired the living room, but when I stayed there, I had flashbacks of how both my body and the house tilted over backward and everything was a mess. I started getting headaches. When there were aftershocks, I couldn't help but cry out.

After the earthquake there was a gasoline shortage, so I could not drive to work. The public buses were always full of passengers, so commuting was hard. Food and gasoline shortages created really long lines when shopping, and there were restrictions on how much we could buy. This made daily life tough. I realized that when I am in a crowd, I always remember these things, and that's why it is so unpleasant. I also realized that I didn't want to admit the difficulty I was having because the damage I suffered was very small compared to people who lost their homes and families. When I realized how I was having difficulty breathing, I was finally able to forgive myself for my own struggles. Then, I was able to calmly remember my own experiences. After three months of yoga therapy, I felt lighter and less tension both mentally and physically. When I didn't have constipation and stiffness in my shoulders anymore, I stopped caring about crowds and could return to a normal life. Now I am regretting how I was defeated by the stress of the earthquake and forgot to be present.

3. Observations

This client had been aware of the importance of practicing yoga therapy, but we think her excessive tension, mental imbalance, and depression resulted from the stress of the earthquake and the fact that she already had a fragile personality. In order to face her own condition, she began using pranayama. She was

Kazuo Keishin Kimura

gradually able to look objectively at her own situation and condition and realized that everyone experiences stress to varying degrees and that it is possible to overcome stress by facing it. When stress is severe, anyone can feel powerless, and trauma can occur. In this case, trauma took root in her mind, but we think that because yoga therapy is able to address the mind, it was helpful in encouraging the development of motivation to face the trauma.

PART IV

Conclusion

CHAPTER 1

Yoga Instruction and Adverse Events

1) The Importance of Yoga Therapy Assessment (YTA)

In modern-day yoga classes, clients are generally not assessed according to traditional yogic principles. I wrote this book with the hope of changing this trend. In conventional medicine, the sciences of anatomy and physiology provide a standard for healthy physical and psychological conditions against which clients are examined, and if there are irregularities, diagnosis is made and treatment is provided in efforts to return clients' conditions to the standard. Compared to conventional medicine, this process is missing in most yoga instruction today. Many people coming to yoga classes have various physical and mental disorders, but instructors are unaware and teach yoga asana, pranayama and meditation techniques without taking their students' conditions into sufficient consideration. Instructors often choose techniques based on their own mood or inspiration at the time, without identifying a clear goal or purpose that has been informed by student's mind-body condition. It is not an overstatement to say that this is the state of modern yoga all over the world.

This is why I wanted to bring more attention to the pancha kosha theory and the human chariot theory, the two theories that are fundamental to yoga therapy. These teachings are expounded upon in ancient scriptures, such as the Upanishads and the *Yoga Sutras*, and have been transmitted over thousands of years by generations of yogis. Based on these scriptures, we have developed several SSIMs that are useful to assess the minds of the clients. I have also introduced some clinical psychology tools.

The reason for placing so much importance on the client's mental condition is because according to traditional yoga, the causes of human suffering are in the functional defects of the buddhi, or the vijnanamaya kosha, which governs human intellect. When the buddhi malfunctions, the functions of the ten sense organs of the manomaya kosha are disturbed, and this in turn disrupts the pranamaya and annamaya kosha functions, leading to the manifestation of disease.

Yoga therapists must, therefore, assess where the vijnanamaya kosha malfunctions when instructing yoga therapy based on this pathogenesis and pathology. Identifying where the intellect has malfunctioned in initial assessments is essential for appropriate and skillful instruction as a yoga therapist.

By receiving yoga therapy instruction, clients themselves can also become aware of where their mental functions have broken down, and discover their own innate ability to heal themselves. To guide clients to "self-healing," yoga therapists must assess the causes of suffering that clients have been unable to identify for themselves—that is, the malfunctions at the vijnanamaya level. Based on these assessments, clients can become aware of the malfunctions, and yoga therapists can provide clients with appropriate practices that empower them to heal themselves and reclaim their health.

2) Yoga Therapy Instruction (YTI) and Changes in the Client's Condition (CCC)

When beginning yoga therapy with a new client, it is important that the yoga therapist first obtains the client's informed consent. After that, the therapist assesses the client's mental and physical condition, and then designs a yoga therapy practice for the client. As the client continues the practice, it is important that the therapist regularly monitors changes in the client's condition (CCC) to ensure that the practice is meeting the client's needs. If the desired CCCs are not confirmed, an assessment should

Yoga Therapy Theory

be done again, with the client's informed consent, and the content of yoga therapy practice should be adjusted accordingly.

To monitor CCC, it is necessary to have objective indicators. For this purpose, we use tools such as POMS, STAI, sVYASA's General Health Questionnaire, and the Japan Yoga Therapy Society's SSIMs during the first few yoga therapy sessions. Then when changes are observed, the same tests can be repeated and the scores compared. Yoga therapists can also use tools from clinical psychology in their efforts to help restore clients to a healthy psychological state.

3) CONCLUSION

This book is an adaptation of a textbook on Yoga Therapy Assessment (YTA) used in a course to train yoga therapists studying to be certified by the Japan Yoga Therapy Society. For yoga instructors and clients, I have tried to keep the explanations relatively simple, though I imagine there may still be many unfamiliar terms. To make yoga therapy available in our modern age for people striving to overcome stress-related disorders, it is necessary to provide explanations of the ancient teachings in terms understood by psychologists, psychiatrists, and medical doctors. Unless we do this, yoga will not be taken seriously, and will be seen only as recreation or exercise at the same level as daily morning stretches.

But yoga is much more than that. From ancient times, seekers traveled to the most remote regions of the Himalayas in search of a guru. Once found, the guru would assess the disciple's mental condition and provide a practice suited to the disciple's mental, physical, and spiritual condition. History has shown us that over decades of practice, an ordinary individual can evolve into a divine being.

I wrote this book based on the principles of human development and evolution extracted from yoga scriptures, as well as the many experiences and realizations I had while receiving direct instruction in traditional yoga from my guru. I am now planning to write a book for medical professionals and clinical psychologists. For students who find what is written in this book to be difficult, refer to the practices for the annamaya kosha in part III, chapter I, and try practicing the yoga therapy techniques in that chapter. If they are hard to understand, I recommend contacting the Japan Yoga Therapy Society. We will introduce you to certified instructors.

I would like to express my gratitude to you for reading to the end of this book. Allow me to finish with a mantra for the happiness and well-being of all living beings.

Sarve bhavantu sukhinah
Sarve santu niramayah
Sarve bhadraani pashyantu
Ma kaschit duhkha bhaag bhaveet
Om shantih, shantih, shantih

May all people be happy
May all people be healthy
May all people enjoy prosperity
May all people overcome suffering
OM peace, peace, peace.

Contact address:
Japan Yoga Therapy Society
1-2-24 Sanbonmatsu
Yonago-shi, Tottori
Japan 683-0842.
Tel: +81-859-22-3503 Fax: +81-859-22-1446
E-mail: yogatherapy@yogatherapy.jp
Website: http://www.yogatherapy.jp/english

ABOUT THE AUTHOR

KAZUO KEISHIN KIMURA WAS BORN in Gunma Prefecture, Japan, in 1947. He graduated from Tokyo University of Education in 1969. After studying for ten years directly under Swami Yogeshwarananda and receiving the holy name Jnana Yogi upon initiation as a Raja Yoga Acharya, Kimura began teaching Raja Yoga. In cooperation with the Swami Vivekananda Yoga Research Foundation, he established and instructed yoga instructor and yoga therapist courses throughout Japan. He is president of the Japan Yoga Therapy Society, executive director of the Japan Integrated Medical Society, and a board member of the Japan Ayurveda Society.

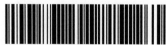

Printed in Germany
by Amazon Distribution
GmbH, Leipzig